Doctors in the Making

Doctors in the Making

Memoirs and Medical Education

Suzanne Poirier

UNIVERSITY OF IOWA PRESS

IOWA CITY

University of Iowa Press, Iowa City 52242
Copyright © 2009 by the University of Iowa Press
www.uiowapress.org
Printed in the United States of America

Design by Sara T. Sauers

The University of Iowa Press is a member of Green Press
Initiative and is committed to preserving natural resources.

Printed on acid-free paper

ISBN-13: 978-1-58729-792-2
ISBN-10: 1-58729-792-2
LCCN: 2008934912

09 10 11 12 13 C 5 4 3 2 1

To my students

Contents

Acknowledgments

I HAVE SPENT my professional years in classrooms, laboratories, and hospital rooms with students and faculty of medicine, nursing, pharmacy, dentistry, and the associated health professions. As a professor of literature in a department of medical education, I have always been aware of the contexts in which I have studied and taught. This book would never have been imagined had we all not shared common concerns about the process and effects of health professionals' education. I began reading and writing about memoirs of medical education soon after coming to work at the University of Illinois at Chicago, but it was a medical student, Bonnie Salomon, who may have first steered me in the direction of this project. She came into my office in the early 1980s to say that the medical students needed a poetry journal—with sizeable cash prizes—to let students know that the emotions had value in medical education. Over the years, several physicians, a nurse, a pharmacist, and an anatomist—Nick Cotsonas, Daniel Brauner, Bill Ahrens, James Wendt, Jay Jacobson, Steve Weine, Ken Simpson, Steve Bergman, Lioness Ayres, Bob Mrtek, and Norman Lieska—have been stalwart teaching companions. They have insisted to students and residents that emotions are important to their humanity as health professionals and have not hesitated to share their own feelings and stories. Outside of medicine entirely, journalism and media scholar Cheryl Koski, through her own development of a typology of autobiographies of medical education, motivated me to return to examining these books in ways different from hers—and I found my path already charted by my excellent students and colleagues.

For over twenty years, the members of the Chicago Narrative and Medicine Reading Group have provided intellectual stimulation and good fun in exploring all the narrative (and then some) dimensions of medical education and practice. In particular, Bill Donnelly's passion for humanistic reform in medical education has kept the plight of medical students and residents always at the center of our minds. I have profited immensely from conversations with innumerable people, but probably most extensively from those with Kathryn Montgomery, Lioness Ayres, Barbara Barzansky, Ilene Harris, Rita Charon, Doug Reifler, Gretchen Case, Dorthea Juul, Barbara Sharf, Anne Hudson Jones, Susan Lawrence, Loreen Herwaldt, Kristi Ferguson, Robert Weir, Sandy Sufian, Sara Vogt, Jonathan Metzl, and Petra Kuppers. Good reading and advice came from Merle Lenihan, Felice Aull, Sayantani DasGupta, Paul John Eakin, and Maura Spiegel. Kate Scannell and Toni Martin steered me to Toni's work. There is no complete bibliography of memoirs of medical education, but I made a good start with Daniel C. Bryant's "Roster of Physician Writers," housed at http://library.med.nyu.edu/library/ eresources/featurecollections/bryant/roster.html. Much of the initial writing of my manuscript was supported by fellowships from the University of Iowa Roy J. and Lucille A. Carver College of Medicine and the Institute for the Medical Humanities, University of Texas Medical Branch. At the University of Iowa Press, Holly Carver, Joe Parsons, and Charlotte Wright have been enthusiastic and helpful from the start, and Gail Zlatnik brought both her head and her heart into pulling my manuscript together.

An earlier version of chapter 3 was published as "Medical Education and the Embodied Physician" in *Literature and Medicine*. My revision here is printed with the permission of the Johns Hopkins University Press. For permission to quote from medschooldiary.com, I thank Emily Baldwin, Brandon Barton, Brian Hartman, Daniel Imler, Marcus Lee, Ron Maggiore, Jamie Taweel, and the Coastal Research Group.

Doctors in the Making

Introduction

I was, I must confess, to lose my temper one day, at a brat I had broken my heart over trying to recondition him. He'd yell at night, every night and only at night, right under my bedroom window across the alleyway, until one night I went to his crib—I could find nothing the matter with him to make him yell—and slapped a piece of three-inch adhesive over his mouth. He could still breathe through his nose, but I thought better of it after a few minutes and took it off again.[1]—WILLIAM CARLOS WILLIAMS

I become less afraid of touching people's hands, of whispering to them in the chaos and bright lights of the Emergency Room. "It's going to be okay," I say quietly, and maybe I'm saying it for them, and maybe I'm saying it for me. Is this playing God? I can't imagine anything further from the truth. . . . We pray that there is another power out there that can heal these people, since it is so clear that the tools we have in our own grasp are painfully, absurdly inadequate.[2]—EMILY BALDWIN

THESE TWO PASSAGES describe events that happened nearly one hundred years apart. William Carlos Williams was in the second year of a residency in pediatrics at Nursery and Children's Hospital in New York City's Hell's Kitchen in 1906. This confession appears in his autobiography, written after more than fifty years of medical practice. In 2002 Emily Baldwin was a third-year medical student at the University of California, San Francisco, when she wrote this entry in her online journal. Although the circumstances and tones of these two excerpts are strikingly different, both offer snapshots of physicians in training at moments of private anguish, moments when they feel that neither compassion nor medicine is sufficient to their patients' needs.

It is important for physicians to learn how to think and act under pressure, but not all pressure is beneficial. Medical education, however well it produces skilled, competent physicians, is a treacherous undertaking for many people. In addition to the demands of school, most medical students and residents are also undergoing their transition into adulthood, a process fraught with its own psychological and emotional hazards. It is unfair to blame medical education for all the angst of those years, but it is also difficult to separate the personal from the professional tasks. Taking adult accountability for one's actions, developing mature political and metaphysical world views, and entering and maintaining relationships within a variety of contexts are also inextricable parts of becoming a humane physician. Going through these developmental processes while working directly with patients ups the proverbial ante associated with the usual work of growing up.

It is the emotional process of becoming a physician that has most engaged my interest in the twenty-five years I have taught medical students, residents, and medical faculty. As a professor of literature in a medical school, working in programs and departments of medical education and medical humanities, I have turned to the printed word to further study this phenomenon. This book is a result of my examination of over forty book-length, personal accounts of medical education published in the United States from 1965 through 2005. Some deal with one or more years of undergraduate medical education (what we most commonly think of as medical school), some with one or more years of graduate medical education (usually called residency), and some span the entire period. Most of them are written within, at most, ten to twelve years of the events related, many within only a few years, and some even within a few hours. These authors write passionately about their experiences, without the buffering or amnesia of a long career. This subjectivity is valuable because it conveys moments that have affected how these young men and women come to view themselves, their patients, and the moral nature of their work. Some experiences give them the strength or affirmation to carry on, and some experiences become defining moments in their professional development.

Medical students and the culture of medical education have long been studied by historians, anthropologists, psychologists, and sociologists. The most thorough history of medical education in the United States is Kenneth M. Ludmerer's two-volume work, *Learning to Heal* and *Time to Heal*, in which he describes the evolution of a medical educational system that harbors longstanding tensions between the biological sciences and clinical medicine, universities and hospitals, and market economics and pedagogy.

Medical sociologists and anthropologists who have studied medical education also tend to study social and cultural structures, but they often add the voices of medical students to their analyses. Early research, most notably Robert K. Merton and colleagues' *The Student-Physician* and Howard S. Becker and colleagues' *Boys in White*, as well as more recent work such as Frederic W. Hafferty's *Into the Valley* and Byron Good's *Medicine, Rationality, and Experience* describe how the structures and values of medicine socialize, reshape, or transform young men and women into physicians. Becker and his colleagues argue that medical education is mostly about learning how to be a student, adopting attitudes that address the particular tensions inherent in the educational process, but Merton and his colleagues speak of a broader notion of *adult socialization*, which extends beyond "education and training" to include "indirect learning, in which attitudes, values, and behavior patterns are acquired as byproducts of contact with instructors and peers, with patients, and with members of the health team."[3] Hafferty also concludes that medical education is part of a larger "resocialization" that generates new "norms about the experience and expression of emotions."[4] Good, examining the cultural nature of medical understanding and practice, describes medical school as a period in which students learn to construct a rational-technical world view, a moral position that also helps them maintain (for themselves even more than for their patients) an emotional stability in the face of fear-evoking situations.[5]

Influential work in narrative, ethnography, and the philosophy of medicine by Kathryn Montgomery, *Doctors' Stories* and *How Doctors Think*, takes the efforts of Becker, Merton, Hafferty, and Good even further. Montgomery demonstrates how the medical profession draws not only on science but also on personal experience (or the personal experience of immediate teachers) in its forms of education and practice. She argues that, while medicine is "scientific," it is "not itself a science,"[6] and she examines the tensions in medical practice between the particularizing nature of caring for individual patients and the generalizing nature of science, between the usefulness and persistence of anecdote or aphorism and an insistence on biomedical evidence, and between the human need for certainty and the inherent uncertainty in the course of many illnesses. She argues that these tensions are seldom addressed in medical education and that the one-sidedness of teaching mostly the scientific aspects of medicine is dangerous and often damaging, not only for its incompleteness but also for its failure to address students' own needs to grapple with the anxieties of medical uncertainty.[7]

More numerous but usually less nuanced are studies of medical education that appear in such journals as *Academic Medicine* and *Medical Education*. A quick survey of these and similar journals beginning with the early 1980s reveals a perennial concern about stress (the term most frequently used) in medical education, particularly in relation to workload, feelings of inadequacy, the emotional experience of death, and the abuse of medical students by faculty.[8] Repeatedly, these researchers found "significant" numbers—ranging from 15 percent to over 50 percent—of students reporting behavior disturbance, depression, anxiety, or disaffection. (Although my study focuses on U.S. medical schools, it is noteworthy that researchers worldwide are publishing similar studies documenting stress in their students and residents.[9]) In more recent years, stress has become such an acknowledged aspect of medical education that medical students are regularly chosen as subjects for studies of the physiological effects of stress.[10] Researchers and educators describe programs designed to reduce the stresses of medical education, such as peer mentors, mental health services, and family services;[11] or courses, usually elective rather than required of all students, in stress management, humanities, wellness, and mindfulness.[12] My cursory review of this literature suggests that more of these kinds of courses than ever before are being introduced into medical schools. As I prepare this manuscript for press, however, my editor has sent me an article from the most recent issue of *Academic Medicine*, "Is There Hardening of the Heart during Medical School?," a question its authors answer in the affirmative, noting that the first and third years of medical school mark the sharpest declines in a measurement called *vicarious empathy*, and that students registering the largest decline choose to go into the more specialized areas of medical practice.[13]

Some medical educators are turning to theories of pedagogy, some originating in fields other than medicine, to address the emotional or reflective development of physicians. In *Educating the Reflecting Practitioner* Donald Schön demonstrates the value of developing greater awareness of one's own thinking processes, particularly in remaining conscious of the steps one takes in performing tasks considered to be automatic once mastered. Lee Shulman, until recently the president of the Carnegie Foundation for the Advancement of Teaching, looks at professional education as an apprenticeship in "cognition" (knowledge), "practice" (skills), and "moral[s]" (integrity).[14] Many family medicine programs have long used self-reflection in small-group discussions as developed and refined by psychologist Michael Balint, in which residents seek to understand their interactions with patients.[15]

In short, I am not alone in my concern about the emotional milieu in which medicine is taught and learned. My study, drawing from resources qualitatively quite different from those of these other scholars, benefits from this breadth of research. Conclusions drawn by scholars in the studies cited above also emerged from my literary analysis of a quite different collection of "data": published *stories* by people scattered across the United States and across more than fifty years. Stories are self-contained accounts in which an author attempts to explain the meaning of an experience, both to him- or herself and to others. Stories can be either fiction or nonfiction and still possess this element of meaning-making. Storytelling is both a personal and a public act: first, the act of writing helps the writer to interpret his or her own life; second, writing to an audience demands that a writer communicate that understanding to readers. Storytelling is, thus, simultaneously reflective and rhetorical.[16]

The writing of nonfiction is, in addition, an exercise in memory. As a writer plumbs her or his memory to fill in the details of an event or characteristics of a person, the emotional impact of that past experience is often revived. This wealth of information, woven together to create a coherent and convincing story, often yields images or subtexts of which a writer may even be unaware. Literary scholars, such as myself, are often more comfortable in the provocative, sometimes elusive realm of stories than we are with measurements or even oral transcripts. We believe that much of understanding is contextual, varies over time, and is often influenced by even the faintest memories or sensations. Literary analysis, however, if not undertaken with close attention to the reader's own predilections and blind spots, can be unreliable—and, although literary scholars often delight in the unreliability of the narrator whose words they study, they must hold themselves accountable for their interpretations. For this reason, in chapter 1, I demonstrate my interpretive style by examining three extended accounts of experiences in emergency medicine.

It is fair, however, to consider how representative are the forty-plus students and physicians who chose to write publicly about their experiences. I have been reassured by the very redundancy of these accounts (a few of them coauthored or "written with" another person), by the predictability of, for example, what kinds of encounters will be described, which situations will cause students the greatest distress or satisfaction, or what qualities are most valued in teachers. Although these memoirs document changes in disease demographics and medical technologies, the causes of grief and joy for the authors remain unchanged over the years. Most students worry about performing successfully almost from the first day of medical school. They report lack of sleep, anxiety about hurting or harming patients, isolation from family and friends, uncertainty about personal involvement with their patients, grief over patients' deaths, and anger about overwhelming amounts of work and the lack of good teaching. There is some vaguely described "loss"—of humanitiy, of idealism, of connection with other people—over the course of medical education, sometimes continuing throughout the years of residency. Chapter 2 presents a description of the tasks and issues that generally arise across the years of medical education.

Even though the accounts that I have examined for this study were written much closer in time to the events than was the story William Carlos Williams told about taping shut his patient's mouth, they still can never exactly capture the raw emotion of a particular moment. As soon as a person puts pen to paper (or fingers to keyboard or, in some instances, voice to tape recorder) a distance opens between author and subject. Choices are made. Doctor X, in *Intern*, the earliest-published book of my study, describes the predicament:

> It is also obvious already that this journal is going to be something different from what I had in mind when I first decided to try to keep it. I had been thinking of recording everything that happened—everything I saw, everything I did, felt or thought, to approach as closely as possible a complete daily record. I can see already that this is ridiculous; there is just too much going on from all sides. There is too much even to remember it to the end of the day, much less get it down on tape. At best I think this is going to be a sporadic diary, dictated by fits and starts in chunks of two or three days at a time if I'm lucky. If I can hit the high spots, get across the things that seem important at the time, and keep it dead honest without pulling any punches, it may still be worthwhile. (17–18)

"Dead honest without pulling any punches" is the stated goal of many of the authors of the stories I have examined, but that doesn't mean that their "honesty" will necessarily be an accurate record of an event. For one thing, as Doctor X observes, "a complete daily record" would be impossible. This may mean that only the best or worst experiences, the kindest or cruelest people, will be remembered. It may also mean that circumstances may be embroidered, others downplayed, in the writers' emotional experiences of those events. There is no such thing as an unmediated story.

All these cautions, however, should merely serve to make me as an interpreter (and each reader, as judge of my interpretation) a more careful reader. I have tried here not to judge the worthiness of a person's anger or the sophistication of a writer's argument. I seek, instead, to discover what causes anger or pleasure; how writers report their reaction to these and other emotions; how medical education might have contributed to these situations and emotional responses; and how medical education might better anticipate, accommodate, and, when possible, alleviate the emotional harshness of medical education.

Physicians and Life Writing

I use the terms *autobiography* and *memoir* interchangeably here, largely because the existing distinctions between these two terms are not consistent. In fact, for some literary scholars, the distinctions have become so blurred that they use the term *life writing* to encompass all prose that purports to be autobiographical in nature. My use of diaries may also be questioned, as some literary conventions are unique to this form of writing. Some scholars of autobiography argue that *any* division between fiction and nonfiction is relative and probably irrelevant, pointing to examples of highly autobiographical fiction and of nonfiction that has been so elaborated upon as to call its veracity into question. Although I tend to be sympathetic to these arguments, I have chosen here to exclude, except in rare instances, any works that identify themselves as fiction, although many of them attest to being thinly veiled autobiography.[17] I do this to make as strong an argument as possible that the texts I study are grounded in the writers' actual experiences.

More significant are the kinds of life writing that I have chosen to exclude: essays about medical education or books in which medical education takes a back seat to practice. By keeping my focus so narrow, I have lost some contributions by people of color, who are already notably underrepresented here. The extra demands often placed on so-called minority physicians or their greater sense of a social-political urgency in their work may militate against the more self-focused exercise of writing memoir. I have also included memoirs only of graduates from medical schools in the United States, for the simple reason that memoirs from other countries do not exist in similar numbers and I want to avoid making false generalizations. In these ways, then, the memoirs considered here may reflect cultural biases, a possibility that I will acknowledge upon occasion throughout this study.

Physicians who have written autobiographies have usually done so within established literary traditions. The form of autobiography probably most familiar to U.S. readers until the last quarter of the twentieth century, the full-life accounting of well-known public figures, has numbered physicians among its contributors from the start, from Benjamin Rush, a signer of the Declaration of Independence, and Elizabeth Blackwell, the first woman to graduate from a U.S. medical school, through other such public figures as S. Josephine Baker, the first head of New York City's Bureau of Child Hygiene, and C. Everett Koop, surgeon general during the administration of Ronald Reagan.[18] For these writers, medical school figures as one or two chapters in a lifetime of medical work. A more specific type of memoir, that of a writer's life and development, counts among its practitioners such U.S. physicians as William Carlos Williams (*The Autobiography of William Carlos Williams*) and Rafael Campo (*The Poetry of Healing*). Physicians have written within the traditions of military and missionary memoir, including such works as, among the former, John A. Parrish's *12, 20, and 5: A Doctor's Year in Vietnam* and Jonathan Kaplan's *The Dressing Station*, and, among the latter, Eva Salber's *The Mind Is Not the Heart* and Thomas A. Dooley's *The Night They Burned the Mountain*. Personal accounts of illness, which have gained popularity in recent decades, have also been written by physicians who became patients: for example, Oliver Sacks (*A Leg to Stand On*); Fitzhugh Mullan (*Vital Signs*); Richard Selzer (*Raising the Dead*); Claudia Osborne (*Over My Head*); and David Biro (*One Hundred Days*). Memoirs that examine only a portion of one's life, usually a period of recent experience, have offered a particularly convenient venue for physicians who treated patients with HIV/AIDS in the early years of the epidemic, such as Abraham Verghese (*My Own Country*), Kate Scannell (*Death of the Good Doctor*), and Peter Selwyn (*Surviving the Fall*). Physicians have written in this form about other unique groups of patients: Lori Arviso Alvord and Elizabeth Cohen Van Pelt about Navajo Indians in New Mexico (*The Scalpel and the Silver Bear*); David Hilfiker about homeless men with HIV/AIDS in Washington, D.C. (*Not All of Us Are Saints*); and Pedro José Greer and Liz Balmaseda about homeless men and women in Miami (*Waking Up in America*). Memoirs about a parent, partner, or close friend have found physician contributors such as Abraham Verghese (*The Tennis Partner*), Peter Selwyn (again, *Surviving the Fall*), and Sherwin Nuland (*Lost in America*). Finally, biomedical science writing, which often portrays the author, although usually not as a fully realized figure, includes such physicians as Oliver Sacks (*The Man Who Mistook His Wife for a Hat*), F. Gonzalez-Crussi (*Notes of an Anatomist*), and Jerome Groopman (*How Doctors Think*). Atul Gawande (*Complications*) and Michael Crichton (*Five Patients*) include their experiences as medical students in their books, but their personal accounts are used more to illustrate broader themes about the limits of medicine and the medical enterprise.

In short, physicians have contributed to all dimensions of autobiographical writing. Conversely, all forms of autobiography possess formats and styles conducive to the expression of medical experiences. That said, I have come to see these nonfiction, extended narratives about medical education as comprising an identifiable subgenre within autobiographical writing.[19] Journalism and media scholar Cheryl A. Koski has gone even further, generating a typology by which to categorize these works.[20] Memoirs about law school exist, but in nowhere near the abundance of memoirs about medical education, as is also true for memoirs about boot camp, perhaps the military equivalent of medical education.

It is significant that the first work that I have identified in this subgenre, *Intern*, by Doctor X, was published in 1965, during a time that what would come to be called investigative reporting was first gaining wide attention. In *Tell Me No Lies* Australian journalist and editor John Pilger defines *investigative reporting* as more than "detective work" and includes within its purview "journalism that bears witness and investigates ideas" (xiv). David L. Protess and his colleagues in journalism, communication, and public affairs refer to investigative reporting as a "journalism of outrage," often advocating agendas of reform. The now-cult novel about residency, *The House of God* by Samuel Shem, published in 1978, sets itself explicitly in the aftermath of Watergate. Both Doctor X and Samuel Shem (also a pseudonym) were highly conscious of the transgressive nature of what they were writing. Doctor X stated his purpose in publishing the journal he kept ten years previously as follows:

> Of course, the profession has not been eager to publicize such incidents, however critical they may be to the education of the doctor-in-training. Such reporting is taboo. . . . People need to understand how a doctor becomes a doctor, what the practice of medicine is all about, what it is that a doctor must put into the game; and, above all, they need some insight into the human limitations upon a doctor's powers. . . .
>
> My intention in publishing this journal has been to contribute to such an understanding between doctors and the general public. (5–6)

Doctor X talks explicitly about needed reforms in his memoir; novelist Shem is more implicit about his goals. His satirical parade of incompetent odd-duck attending physicians, self-protective and sometimes sociopathic residents, and irreverent rebellious interns is, nevertheless, a cry of outrage against residency training, one that continues to generate commentary more than thirty years later.[21]

The tone sounded in both *Intern* and *The House of God* reverberates throughout many of the medical memoirs and novels that have been published subsequently. They continue to tell the proverbial stories out of school, both to bring the secrets of medicine—one hopes—to the cleansing and healing light of day and to paint a human picture of physicians for the public. Twenty years later, David Hellerstein echoed Doctor X almost exactly, although seemingly without the same rancor:

> Patients often write about their experiences; *doctors, trained in silence*, rarely do. However, by writing about a world that is commonly misunderstood and misrepresented, one can show the realities of life better than through a thousand surveys or questionnaires. A doctor who writes can complete the picture, can show not only the extent of problems and miscommunications between doctor and patient, the paradoxes, the confusions and incongruities along with the victories and small miracles, but can also open the possibility of finding solutions. (10, my italics)

At the same time that these authors express goals similar to those of investigative reporters, they often write about the benefits *to themselves* of writing about their experiences. Charles LeBaron, author of *Gentle Vengeance*, one of the first memoirs about undergraduate medical education (in fact about only his first year of medical school) sounds a theme of self-understanding that is heard throughout many of these books:

> It seemed to me I had a little vial of sweetness and kindness around stomach level. It'd been full when I was born . . . but I was hanging on for dear life to those remaining couple ounces. They had me for six or so more years, ample chance to make me spill the rest in wrath or discouragement.
>
> If I were to lead a life free of the influences they seemed determined to inflict on me, if I were ever to exact that gentle vengeance, it would require some extraordinary stability in my internal environment. . . . Writing a book about those influences and the experiences they created might help me maintain some detachment, give me an objectivity, an independence, where none might otherwise exist. (268–69)

Perri Klass, a published writer of fiction before she began medical school who was invited to write about her experiences for various publications throughout the years of her medical education, saw her essays as a record of the person she must necessarily leave behind:

> The experience of writing about medical school while going through it has changed my medical education tremendously. I have found that in order to write about my training so that people outside the medical profession can understand what I am talking about I have had to preserve a certain level of naiveté for myself. . . .
>
> The general pressure in medical school is to push yourself ahead into professionalism, to start feeling at home in the hospital, in the operating room, to make medical jargon your native tongue. . . . You want to leave behind that green, terrified medical student who stood awkwardly on the edge of the action, terrified of revealing limitless ignorance, terrified of killing a patient. . . .
>
> The essays in this book were written during the four years I spent in medical school. . . . I have not altered these pieces to make them more uniform, because it seems to me that if my voice has changed through medical school, then that change should be part of the education process I have been writing about.[22]

Several of the authors of these memoirs describe writing as both a way of preserving a part of oneself and a means of better understanding an emotionally overwhelming situation. Using writing as, itself, a way of coping with the stresses of medical school may make these memoirists unique. Other students and physicians may find outlets more suited to their talents and interests. I shall say more about storytelling in medical education in the conclusion.

Finally, the proof that memoirs of medical education have succeeded in establishing their own subgenre resides in the literary begats that have sprung up among the forty-plus memoirs that have been published since 1965. Titles themselves tell the tale, with William Nolen's *The Making of a Surgeon* in 1968 followed by David S. Viscott's *The Making of a Psychiatrist* (1972), Elizabeth Morgan's *The Making of a Woman Surgeon* (1980), Claire McCarthy's *Learning How the Heart Beats: The Making of a Pediatrician* (1995), and Craig A. Miller's *The Making of a Surgeon in the Twenty-first Century* (2004). Authors themselves, particularly after 1990, began citing one or more memoirs in their own writing. For example, Miller (*The Making of a Surgeon*

in the Twenty-first Century) cites Nolen's *Making of a Surgeon* (214), and Sayantani DasGupta (*Her Own Medicine,* this title itself an allusion to Abraham
Verghese's *My Own Country*) mentions Perri Klass's *A Not Entirely Benign
Procedure* (6). Bloggers Emily Baldwin and Ron Maggiore report encounters
with physician-writers Abraham Verghese and John Stone (a poet whose
work is not included here), evidence that physician-writers are known to
many of these authors.[23] Michael Greger displays the most extensive awareness of memoirs of medical education in *Heart Failure,* the heavily annotated
journal of his third year of medical school, in which he cites, among others,
Philip Reilly, Michelle Harrison, Melvin Konner, Samuel Shem, Perri Klass,
and Charles LeBaron. Although most of these memoirs have received little
critical acclaim and are not widely known, they are taken seriously by their
readers. As I have spoken to medical students over the years, I have learned
that many of them have read at least one of these books. Even with a relatively small readership, presses, several of them quite prestigious, continue
to publish these books on a regular basis. Because the content of these texts
is of greater importance to my study than the gracefulness of literary styles,
much of their individuality will be lost in the chapters that follow. In each
chapter, however, I provide at least one longer excerpt from a memoir that
will more fully bring a writer's unique voice to readers.

Storytellers and Their Stories

Although medical school follows a strictly ordered sequence of courses, chronology alone does not make a story. Broadly stated, a story interprets events,
even chooses which events to tell with a particular interpretation in mind. The
advance of time, however, is crucial in stories of medical education, because
the curriculum of medical education is arranged so sequentially. Probably for
this reason most writers of memoirs of medical education adopt a narrative
structure that emphasizes a linear chronology. The fictional form that lends
itself well to the adventures of physicians in training is the *picaresque,* literally
the story of a rogue, most often a "retelling of . . . adventures in the service of
a series of masters," whose cleverness (sometimes criminality) pits him or her
against a society that deserves mockery or satire. Famous *pícaros* of literature
include Don Quixote, Moll Flanders, and Huckleberry Finn.[24] Less given
to satire is the *Bildungsroman,* a form of German origin, whose subject is the
development, often the education, of a (usually) young person, particularly
his or her philosophical and moral development. Goethe's *Wilhelm Meister's*

Apprenticeship is the model for this genre, which also includes such works as Charles Dickens's *David Copperfield* and Thomas Mann's *The Magic Mountain.*²⁵ More modest in scope than the *Bildungsroman* but similar in intent is what is usually called the coming-of-age story, in which a young person discovers that a revered elder (often a parent or teacher) or one's idyllic world is flawed. William Faulkner's "Barn Burning" and Alice Walker's "To Hell with Dying" are frequently anthologized stories in this mode. All of these plot lines are utilized by the writers of the memoirs I examine here, in part because these time-honored stories *do* represent archetypal patterns that are echoed in the process of medical education: a rogue resident meets stock representations of medical greed, coldness, or monomania; the frightened, green medical student comes, through his or her mistakes and heartbreaks, to find self-assurance and renewed compassion for patients; and, repeatedly, idealistic students and residents find that the very profession of medicine stands metaphorically on feet of clay. Also, though, these familiar narrative structures may be adopted unconsciously by novice writers, who may not fully realize the rhetorical or moral stance inherent in these forms. It is well to remember that memoirs of medical education reflect the structures of literature as well as of memory.

Whatever the form, most of these stories depend on the presence of a main character. Although many of these authors would be reluctant to characterize themselves as heroic, they often adopt a stance that places them in conflict with the actions or values of their teachers, other students, the healthcare or educational systems within which they work, and, at times, even their patients. At the same time, they often picture themselves as damaged by their experiences. They may better fit the definition of existential hero or antihero, a character that also corresponds with the times in which this subgenre emerged. Whether hero or antihero, however, this central figure is imbued with generations of literary tradition. In the United States the "American hero" has a unique political and literary history. Early observers, such as Alexis de Tocqueville and Hector St. John de Crèvecoeur, described the citizens of this new nation as particularly individualistic and self-reliant, characteristics that de Tocqueville also warned could lead to an individual's isolation from other people.

More recently, Robert N. Bellah and his colleagues explored the notion of individualism as it has evolved in the United States. They remarked, among other things, that this individualism has been so taken as an emblem of *citizens* of the U.S. that people often overlook the equally prominent role that citizen*ship* played in that young society—a *communal* identity that has been as central as individualism in the country's development from its earliest days. Bellah and his colleagues offer the literary figures of the cowboy and the private detective as exemplars of a quintessential American hero: a singular man who can shoot "faster and straighter" than anyone else; defends society against ill-doing and injustice, often at considerable cost to himself; and yet is a loner, kept from joining the rest of humankind because of his special skills and mission.[26] In *The American Adam*, R. W. B. Lewis describes the articulation of a national identity that valorized the man (almost without exception a man) who was self-reliant, brave, ingenious, and a protector of the unfortunate. Usually a loner in a discomforting or even hostile society, his innocence is assaulted by the evil around him, and his self-assurance is put to the test. He is often damaged in the process but usually emerges wiser and stronger—and wiser and stronger than those around him.[27]

This national heroic identity was becoming enmeshed with cultural values and social mores at the same time that medical educators in the United States were seeking to establish training programs that could compete with the European centers of medical education, most notably France and Germany.[28] Medicine, entering the age of microbiology and germ theory, was gaining a reputation for new (curative) power, and experimental science was being hailed as the new frontier for medicine. These physicians longed to be seen as its leading pioneers. The aspirations of U.S. academic physicians and the popular imagination of the country's citizens converged in the first part of the twentieth century to create an archetypal physician-hero: Martin Arrowsmith of Sinclair Lewis's novel *Arrowsmith*. Brilliant, dashing, daring, self-sacrificing, yet humble, Martin Arrowsmith shows particular talents for scientific research, a path he follows haltingly at first, nearly defeated by the greed and glamour of the physicians, scientists, and politicians he meets along the way. Eventually, chastened by his own overreaching, Arrowsmith sees the falseness of those around him, forsakes the trappings of wealth and fame, and removes himself, with just the basics of his laboratory equipment, to a secluded workshop in the woods. However exaggerated, even melodramatic, the depiction of Dr. Arrowsmith may seem today, his image pervades the popular media. Even the flawed doctor-heroes of television and film in recent years manage to fight for the underdog, miraculously save the sick more often than not, usually know better than their superiors and prove those people wrong at whatever cost to themselves, and exhibit superior moral wisdom or courage however rough their manners.[29]

Although medical schools do not promote heroism as a set of explicit behaviors, medical curricula overwhelmingly advocate creating physicians who are self-reliant, uniquely accountable for their actions, and self-sacrificing. These qualities are important in a physician, but they also echo a mythic vision of young American manhood that may have been flawed, or at least incomplete, at its outset. Tellingly, it is this image of the lone, self-sufficient, heroic physician that most U.S. memoirists, men as well as women, find most problematic as they move through their years of medical education.

It wasn't until quite far along in my study that I realized that I had uncovered no memoirs of medical education by Canadian students or physicians, although as I wrote the final draft of this manuscript Vincent Lam had been awarded Canada's Scotiabank Giller Prize for his collection of short fiction, *Bloodletting and Miraculous Cures*, which follows a set of recurring characters from premed days into medical practice. As fiction, the work would not qualify for my study, but it may signal an opening door for physician-memoirists in Canada. This absence may simply reflect the larger number of publishing houses in the United States or the effects on medical education of a different health system. Although Canadian medical schools are generally considered more innovative in their curricula than U.S. schools, Canadian curriculum reforms adopted by U.S. schools, as portrayed in several of the memoirs, do not seem to alleviate students' anxieties or complaints. One Canadian study suggests that, whatever the curriculum, Canadian students report "manageable" levels of stress, unlike the majority of most studies of U.S. students.[30] These studies are hardly sufficient to conclude that different national settings equate to different levels of stress in medical education, but they raise provocative questions about national cultures and professional development.

Studies of medical education that have their roots in the sociology and anthropology of professions often use terms such as *socialization, ritual, initiation,* and *rite of passage* to describe the adoption of a professional identity. Becker and colleagues, for example, characterize medical education as "one of the longest rites of passage in our part of the world" (4). Anthropologist Victor Turner is probably best known for his exploration of these concepts. In his influential *Dramas, Fields, and Metaphors,* Turner writes about the "social dramas" by which a cultural group continues to define itself. He finds grist for his ethnographic mill in such diverse subjects as religious practices, historical events, and cultural groups ranging from the Ndembu of Africa to the hippies of Haight-Ashbury. Expanding on the earlier work of Arnold ven Gennep, Turner characterizes rites of passage as having three stages: separation, liminality, and reaggregation.

The second phase interests him most. *Liminality*, Turner writes, is a period in the ritual process in which the person undergoing the rite of passage

> becomes ambiguous, neither here nor there, betwixt and between all fixed points of classification; he passes through a symbolic domain that has few or none of the attributes of his past or coming state. . . . In liminality, the symbolism almost everywhere indicates that the initiand . . . is structurally if not physically invisible in terms of his culture's standard definitions and classifications. He has been divested of the outward attributes of structural position, set aside from the main arenas of social life in a seclusion lodge or camp, and reduced to an equality with his fellow initiands regardless of their preritual status. (232)

My own reading confirms that liminality is a state experienced by medical students—and even residents—throughout many years of their education. Young adults who enter medical school enter a state in which participants are not yet doctors but are no longer laypersons or *nonphysicians* (a telling term, really, when one considers that most of the world is made up of nonphysicians). Almost from the minute they are accepted into medical school, they are granted the status and many of the accompanying privileges of doctors, a lie that causes many students discomfort, even though they desire the knowledge and skill that designation implies. Conversely, physicians even at the end of their residency often report their dismay when patients or established physicians do not recognize that they *are* now licensed physicians, at the same time that many of them also admit anxieties about leaving the shelter of their residency programs. During these years, students and residents both seek and fear an identity that their teachers, their families, and society at large demand of and deny them.

Chapters 3 through 5 show the medical student or resident struggling, from this liminal position, to understand three dilemmas of medical practice that are seldom addressed in their curricula: physical vulnerability, power, and relationship. In each of these chapters, I draw evidence both across the memoirs and within selected texts, the former by a series of short quotations from several memoirs and the latter by closer readings of a few, longer passages. The more-numerous short quotations support the generalizability of the experiences I describe, and the lengthier excerpts allow a fuller examination of the complexity of the issues the writers present.

One distinctive feature of these memoirs is the delight all the authors seem to take in regaling their readers with the most graphic, raw descriptions, not only of patients but of their own physical condition. Examination of these passages, however, led me to decide that they are usually a reflection of the writers' discomfort with the physical intimacy inherent in their work. Usually beginning with the first day in gross anatomy lab, smell and touch, with imagined taste hovering always nearby, join sight and sound in the experience of medical education and practice. Sleeplessness, hours of standing in surgery, and the feel of a patient's blood gone cold and clammy when soaked into an intern's clothes make medicine a profession that marks the bodies of its practitioners. The vulnerability that such embodiment teaches medical students is the subject of chapter 3, in which I argue that medical education should attend to the physical well-being of its protégés far more than it has done in the past.

In chapter 4 I examine the various dynamics created by cultural differences and the role of power in both medical education and the practice of medicine. The long history in the U.S. of physicians being primarily white Protestant men establishes many grounds for cultural and economic difference—and, consequently, tension or miscommunication—between physicians and patients. As the medical profession itself has become more diverse, issues of difference have appeared among physicians themselves, with differences in gender the most thoroughly documented in these memoirs. The close connections between socioeconomic status, education, and power also create a divide between physicians and patients, whatever other cultural differences might exist. Medical education, however, and the liminal state in which it places students and residents creates another differential: physicians in training often reach points in the course of their education when they feel even less powerful than their patients. In such a state, students and residents can become disrespectful, even abusive, of the patients in their care. It is an illogical response, which most of the writers realize, but it demonstrates dramatically the complex nature of power in the work of physicians.

Both men and women report situations in which their actions, ones that they often regret, are born out of their sense of isolation, anxiety, and helplessness. In these instances, authors write gratefully about those physicians who acknowledge their students' feelings and help them through such emotionally difficult times. They also write at length about the patients who evoke strong reactions in them, both positive and negative. The term most used to discuss *connection* with patients is, ironically, *distance*, a word meant to connote the position in which a physician can offer both compassion and sound medical judgment. These instances often belie the image of the objective, self-sufficient physician. By far the largest part of these memoirs addresses the authors' struggles to establish comfortable, workable, and fulfilling relationships with their patients, teachers, peers, and friends and family. The memoirs abound with stories of the countless kinds of relationships in which medical students and physicians engage daily, and authors repeatedly express a desire for greater connection with the people around them. In chapter 5 I explore these writers' depiction of medicine as a relational profession and consider how that reconceptualization might lead us to rethink some of the goals of medical education.

In the conclusion, I turn to the medical curriculum itself, a leviathan that is remarkably similar from one medical school to another, in which change *does* occur, but often very gradually. Even with the addition, over the past few decades, of courses in patient-physician communication, medical ethics, and professionalism, medical curricula still fail to respond to the emotional needs of many of their students. Drawing upon these memoirs, I shall offer some suggestions for ways to redress the vaguely defined inhumanity of medical education. My recommendations are seemingly modest, calling primarily for emotional honesty as a pedagogical precept throughout all the years of medical education. It could be practiced easily, but its longtime absence from medical education—and in the professed culture of medical practice itself—makes it a greater challenge than creating a new course in the already overfull curriculum.

In writing a book about what is wrong with medical education, it is easy to misrepresent my own viewpoint. So it bears repeating: the job of producing competent, conscientious physicians is a demanding and difficult task, and, for the most part, schools and colleges of medical education succeed in doing so. There are good teachers as well as bad ones, although the latter fill more pages in the memoirs. It is too easy to blame all the ills of medical education on a cumbersome, impersonal educational or healthcare "system" that damages students and teachers alike. I don't want to absolve physicians and students of all unkind thoughts or deeds. However, an overextended, usually underfunded system allows teachers and students alike to avoid confronting and working through difficult emotions and relationships. Demanding schedules and lack of time can offer ready excuses for not sparing a few minutes for self-reflection or to support a grieving student.

Most physicians will say that their education was difficult, often grueling, but most of them survive its rigors and go on to practice, happily, the profession to which many aspired from their youth. Nevertheless, many students suffer severe emotional distress during the process of their education, distress that is not proven to be necessary or even beneficial. At its worst, patients also suffer the effects of a student's or resident's anxiety or anger. Some physicians feel that they have sacrificed an important part of their identity in the process of becoming a doctor, a part of themselves, moreover, that might have made them a more caring physician, spouse, or colleague. They mourn these losses, and some of them turn to writing to bear witness to this loss. In their writing, they seek to become whole again. The final lesson that these memoirs of medical education may teach is the power of life writing as a tool for maintaining, even developing, emotional wholeness—a skill that might be as important for young physicians to learn as drawing blood or tying sutures.

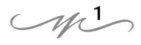

Voices from the Emergency Room

USING LITERARY WORKS as a source of data for research poses particular challenges. Whenever we read or hear a story, we inevitably form impressions about the characters and their actions. Those impressions are based on our own, unique experiences, likes and dislikes, values, even the mood we're in at the time.[1] As a scholar, I must monitor my personal response to these stories to make sure it isn't overriding my critical judgment. I also need to convince readers that the way I interpret these stories is reasonable and that the conclusions I draw from them are conclusions that other careful readers might reach as well.

For these reasons, one purpose of this chapter is to demonstrate my interpretive process. To do this, I have chosen three accounts set in emergency rooms. Choosing one setting provides a constant across stories that vary in time, age of the narrator, and narrative form and style. In the years between the early 1950s and early 2000s emergency medicine became a formal specialty with its own certifying examinations, residency programs, and professional journals. Residency training in emergency medicine takes place not only in emergency rooms but also on surgical floors and intensive care units. Indeed, even before it was its own field, much of emergency medicine involved not only one-time encounters with patients, but also what is called followup, tracking the course of a patient's care through recovery or return visits to a hospital's clinics.[2]

In the three accounts quoted below, I provide larger excerpts than will appear in later chapters and talk about the longer works from which they are drawn, so that readers can observe how I place my analysis within the context of a full work. Even this close look at a few, specific memoirs, however, introduces most of the ideas that I shall examine more closely in subsequent chapters. Whatever the differences in the literary aspects of these three works, the concerns that the writers express about their patients, their colleagues, and themselves suggest a consistency that transcends time, place, and personality. Thus, a second purpose for this chapter is to introduce themes that will recur throughout this study.

A third purpose is to introduce readers to the range of styles these memoirs take. As literary works, these memoirs of medical education are of particular interest to me in terms of their narrative form and voice. The three works I consider here—private diary, traditional memoir, and electronic blog—place their narrators in different kinds of relationships not only with their readers but also with their subject matter. Authors choose stances that place greater or lesser distance between themselves as creators, narrators, and actors in their life stories. For a critical reader, it is important to attend to how literary devices affect the kinds of stories that writers craft. As an examiner of medical education in this undertaking, I need to be mindful of how literature works—and works *on* me—if my judgments are to reflect the *content* of the memoirs and not their style.

With this orientation to these memoirs comes an additional caveat: as a professor of literature and not medicine, I do not attempt to judge the accuracy or wisdom of any of the medical diagnoses or decisions reported by these authors. Although, particularly for the patients involved, this is an important consideration, my concern here is with the process of medical education itself. Hopefully, attention to the latter will eventually benefit the former as well.

Theodore Isaac Rubin, circa 1952

In the 1950s, Theodore Isaac Rubin kept a diary of the last four months of his internship, during his rotation (the term for the various clinical specialities to which students and residents are assigned) in the emergency room of a nonprofit community hospital in southern California. Rubin did not publish the diary until nearly twenty years later, motivated, he says, by the similarities he heard in his own son's accounts of internship. "There are some new lab tests and medical advances," Rubin writes, "but responsibility for people in every conceivable kind of medical difficulty is the same now as it was then."[3] By 1972, Rubin was a practicing psychoanalyst and the president of the American Institute for Psychoanalysis. His fictionalized case study, *Lisa and David* (1961), one of several such novels he published between 1960 and 1965, had been made into an acclaimed film. He was a regular columnist in the *Ladies' Home Journal* and the author of a number of self-help books in the area of mental health. Five years later, he would publish a memoir of his recent practice, *Reflections in a Goldfish Tank*, also written in diary form.

Thus, although *Emergency Room Diary* was published seven years after *Intern*, it probably documents the earliest period within my study of this genre. Rubin claims that the diary is unaltered from its original writing, thus making it an almost daily record of his immediate experiences. He writes in the preface,

> Re-reading my diary of that time makes me feel a bit embarrassed by the somewhat unsophisticated young man who lived it—but I feel rather satisfied with him too. Those four months and the following year of weekends in the E.R. made a deep and lasting impression. I feel that my E.R. time, more than anything else during that period of my life, contributed to personal growth, a sense of professional responsibility, and the ability to make decisions. This all sounds rather ponderous, but it is nevertheless true. The E.R. did a fast and remarkably thorough job, in the short time I spent there, of ridding me of many childish illusions regarding the human condition, more specifically those involving medicine, doctors, and myself. It also helped prepare me for future confrontations. There have been many things that have fazed me since those days, but I've not been nearly as shook up or vulnerable as I might have been without the E.R. experience. In short, it was invaluable in helping me to grow up, humanly and professionally—and of course there is no dichotomy there. Both are part of the same process. (vii–viii)

Although Rubin does not say that his diary is reprinted verbatim, his admission to being embarrassed by his earlier self implies that he has allowed his account to retain what he was thinking and doing during that period in his life. "The facts are true," he avers. "All of it has happened" (viii). Every literary scholar, however, is cautious around such proclamations of authenticity. Very few authors can move directly from raw text into print without editing themselves, so it is hard to believe that a diary, especially one written in the rush of an internship, would remain completely unaltered. At the very least, grammar, punctuation, and some syntax have probably been changed, as the prose reads with a smoothness that might not occur in the press of daily writing. Once a person is cleaning up a manuscript, there is always the possibility of filling in a sketchy entry or deleting a passage. And there is always the chance that *Emergency Room Diary* is not a diary at all, but merely crafted to sound impulsive and immediate. As a reader, I can allow myself to be swept away, but as a commentator on medical education, I need to feel assured that what I am reading is a conscientious, honest reporting of individual experiences.

Rubin makes a special effort to separate his dual role as original author and subsequent presenter of his diary. As the *presenter* of *intern* Ted Rubin, *author* Theodore Isaac Rubin writes a preface in which he comments that he has "not named the place and . . . [has] changed the names of the people for obvious reasons" (viii). In an introduction he establishes the general setting of the diary, describes how an emergency room functions, sketches the structure of the residency program in intern Ted Rubin's hospital, provides the names (invented, as he says, except for his own) and brief sketches of the people who will appear in the diary, and explains the equipment, drugs, and the most common procedures used in the emergency room of his internship. He follows the diary with a glossary, "Emergency Room Medical Terms and Hospital Jargon."

These supplements permit the diary itself to begin *in medias res*, with the reader immediately immersed in the life of intern Ted Rubin. No dates are given to the entries, creating the sense of hurried notes, some brief and some long, some reportorial and some editorial. This format is similar to the style of his writing in his fictional case stories, suggesting not only that he may have adapted this episodic, quasi-stream-of-consciousness mode to a variety of forms, but also that he favors an informal, emotionally expressive persona as the narrator of his stories. Below are the first five entries in Rubin's diary, written in the early 1950s:

Today a new doctor came on duty. He's about fifty years old, short, bulky, toothy, and very clumsy—all in all, rather sloppy looking, too. We were introduced. His name is Waggoner, and his English is four-fifths German. He's doing an internship so that he can get a license here in California. I can't resist and I ask him, and he tells me. Yes, he was a member of the Nazi party. Through no fault of his own and all the rest of the no-fault apologetic crap: he had to join or he couldn't practice, etc. Me, Ted Rubin—a Jew—I listen to all this politely, like I understand and accept it all. So there we are: me a Jew and him a Nazi making like a doctor, pretending we dig each other so nicely. It's disgusting. I don't mean him—I mean me. I ought to walk out or at least ignore him or something. Instead, I find I want to believe him, all the stuff about his not being able to help it and that he did no harm and all the rest of that garbage. God, how half-assed I am. Why don't I spit in his eye or something? Is it cowardice? I'm half his age and twice his size! Even as I write this, I begin to feel sorry for him. Me and this crazy self-effacing Jewish nobility of mine. Morgan wants me to help acquaint him with things. Instead of kicking his ass, I'll wind up mothering him. A Nazi, no less. It's unbelievable!

Waggoner couldn't have done too much damage—he's too dumb. But so were a lot of the other bastards who worked the gas chambers.

He really knows from shit, though. I wonder whether he had anything at all to do with medicine before he came here. . . . He gave an asthmatic woman I.V. aminophyllin today in ten seconds flat. Also, he forgot to take the tourniquet off before injecting the stuff. This guy will kill somebody for sure if he's not watched!

We had eighty-eight cases today. A record for the week—so far. There are three of us, but I swear I saw seventy of the eighty-eight. I'm so tired I can't move. Funny, me calling them cases! Just a few months ago I made big lectures to myself to remember that *people* must never become *cases* if I'm ever to become a decent psychiatrist when I leave here.

I'm so tired I feel drugged. I'm nauseated from it—or from eating so damn much. These twenty-four-hour stints will kill me for sure. Not the work or the fatigue, but the food: the more tired I am, the more I eat. Christ, I'm up to 251. I've got to get myself impressed with the lunacy of this or I'll eat my way into an infarct for sure. Can't wait to begin psychiatry. But have to admit this E.R. work gives me a good feeling, too. No more hamburgers, though—I solemnly swear, as of tomorrow A.M. proper dieting stat!

It took Waggoner four hours to suture a leg laceration today. The woman was so stiff from lying in one spot she couldn't straighten up when we took her off the table. . . . It was a long cut—from her knee to her ankle—but no tendons, arteries, or complications. Should have taken half an hour at most. Four hours—I clocked him. Fifty-year-old Nazi—maybe he would have liked to butcher her instead. That's not nice. But, who's nice and why?

Today a sixty-year-old man came in with a huge prostate in severe urinary retention. His belly was as big as a nine-month pregnancy. I just couldn't pass the catheter. But I learned something—me, the would-be psychiatrist.

I called the urologist, Dr. Robert Jason, and he straightened me out—and the patient, too. I was all set for a cystotomy or something else fancy and complicated. But Dr. Jason gave him some Seconal and 100 mg. of Demerol and put him in a side room for half an hour. He then had me pass the catheter, easy as pie. Just a little time, sedation, and relaxation make all the difference in the world. A good lesson that I won't forget! (23–26)

The reader's first encounter with the written voice of intern Ted Rubin is a rant about a new intern: an older, immigrant physician who was a member of the Nazi party in Germany, who must spend a year as an intern before qualifying to take the examination needed to practice medicine in the U.S. Waggoner's presence dominates the early pages of Rubin's diary, as does Rubin's disgust with having to work alongside him—and his disgust with himself for politely doing so. Although Waggoner tells him that he was not a willing member of the party and did not participate in any of the atrocities of the Holocaust, Rubin still often equates him with those activities: "dumb . . . [like] a lot of the other bastards who worked the gas chambers" and "maybe he would have liked to butcher her instead." Rubin uses his diary to air his anger at having to work with Waggoner, but the process of writing also puts him into an immediate dialogue with himself, in which a more reasonable person hears the angry intern's words. "Even as I write this, I begin to feel sorry for him," he says in his first entry. In the fourth entry, his two voices argue with each other, with the angry voice permitted the last word: "butcher her instead. That's not nice. But, who's nice and why?"

Two aspects of this passage are of particular interest to me. The first is that of relationships and the writer's attempt to understand and manage them. The learning and practice of medicine require a constant juggling of relationships that are, themselves, constantly shifting in the busy, often anxiety-ridden settings in which undergraduate and graduate medical education occur. When we think of physicians' relationships, it is most often (and appropriately) with patients, but these memoirs also show the writers struggling to establish comfortable relationships with colleagues and peers, teachers and supervisors, and even their own friends and families.

Rubin's ongoing struggle to accommodate Waggoner within his world is one of the more dramatic relationships portrayed in these memoirs, but Rubin also talks about his relationships with other people, including nurses, attending physicians, and patients. Patients actually receive much more attention in his journal than his first entries suggest. Take the following, for example, from about halfway through the diary:

> Just can't get over the fact that Mrs. James is dead. I guess I convinced myself that she was going to make it. With minimal anastomosis around the heart, people under fifty have so much less chance of making it than older people with infarcts.
>
> Sailor's legs are warm! Please God, he shouldn't blow an embolus or anything crazy!

> Was thinking about life and death and the whole lousy bit. Mrs. James again. Had a muddled dream about her that I can't remember. Hope L.U.P. and Sailor make it. In my dream there was something about Madden's pulmonary embolus case, too. I guess psychiatrists can have pretty rough times, too, deciding whether or not a guy is dangerous or suicidal and should or shouldn't be hospitalized. I suppose I'm just feeling tired and morbid. It's not all fun and games, and the good guys don't always win. (96–97)

Mrs. James is still on Rubin's mind several weeks later, when he despairs over another patient: "Dreamed of Johnson's Poor machine woman last night and cried in my sleep. Why? I hardly knew her. This is one whom I'm sure I felt and feel relatively detached from. Maybe she reminded me of Mrs. James. Jesus—psychiatry should be a welcome haven from all this lousy maiming and dying!" (147). Rubin writes about the tension between detachment and involvement that all the memoirists frequently describe. Even when one deliberately seeks detachment, however, it is often not possible.

The second aspect of interest to me is that of writing, particularly reflective writing, as a useful tool in a physician's professional and personal development. Keeping this diary has allowed Ted Rubin to, in a sense, talk to himself throughout this period. Not all of his writing is reflective, however; much of it could more accurately be called reactive, blowing off steam or indulging in self-pity. It is possible, though, that the very process of writing, versus stewing on a walk or train ride home, provides a mental—and even physical—space for thoughts to be seen, examined, and responded to in a more measured manner. In Ted Rubin's diary the reflective process is so fluid at times it becomes stream-of-consciousness. The style of this reflection is one reason why I believe this book to be an actual diary (or drawn largely verbatim from an existing diary). It is a pattern that would require considerable skill to insert with such naturalness twenty years after the fact.

Many of the memoirs offer their most reflective thinking at the end of a chapter or the book itself. These reflections usually take a broader look at how the author feels he or she has developed as a physician, and they usually note, with some amazement, an achieved degree of comfort and confidence in one's role. Rubin engages in this type of reflection at the close of his diary, in a voice that is characteristically self-questioning, even with his new sense of assurance:

> Being on twenty-hour days for nearly a week, practically alone, has left me no thinner than before. I'm back to 250 again. But it has given me a certain confidence—confidence and $60 [Rubin has taken a part-time job in a neighboring emergency room during the last weeks of his four months on E.R. rotation]. I'm pretty good at this E.R. thing. I really believe I actually did much of it sleepwalking. Anyway, it gives me a sense of accomplishment that feels very good. I've got more stamina than I thought. I know it's pretty silly and childish, but it does make me feel a little heroic. I suppose it sort of fits in with the kid fantasies I used to have of being the self-sacrificing doctor and all that. Horney's neurotic glory? Maybe, but also a feeling of what I suspect is genuine self-satisfaction, that I hope I can go on owning in the future. Maybe this is pretty damn arrogant on my part, but I'm really beginning to think that I've discovered my second big talent. The first, which I discovered in medical school, was a genius for gin rummy—which is boring and useless. This, the second, may be E.R. work—which I suppose will be useless also. I just hope the third turns out to be psychiatry. (143–44)

The tone of lightly humorous self-deprecation, with an overlay of bravado, is the same one we heard in the opening entries of the diary, but it is more measured here. In part, an end-of-rotation reflection prompts a more formal, deliberately thoughtful report, but we still hear the voice of a young physician enthralled and somewhat intimidated by the world he is preparing to enter. But he's willing to proclaim himself better prepared for what might come. Ted Rubin does not possess the breadth of understanding of what he's been through that Theodore Rubin assesses twenty years later, but the intern clearly knows that he is more sure of himself in ways both professional and personal than he was four months earlier.

In addition to the presence of Dr. Waggoner, another event during these months made Rubin acutely aware of being Jewish. Early in the rotation, Rubin learns from the hospital's business manager, Mr. Quistle, that he will not receive the year-end bonus of one thousand dollars awarded to all English-speaking interns. *English-speaking*, it turns out, really means physicians who trained in U.S. medical schools. Rubin attended medical school in Lausanne, Switzerland, as did a significant number of Jewish Americans at that time, their entrance into U.S. medical schools limited by a very restrictive quota system.[4] Rubin rails against the discriminatory double whammy: "I feel took! Discriminated against! Prejudiced against! Like a second-class citizen! I feel like saying fuck you, and walking out of this lousy place. Why the hell did I come here to California anyway? These dirty duplicitous sons of bitches" (29).

Rubin's rancor continues through the four months of the diary, although he usually talks about it in terms of the thousand-dollar bonus that is denied him (no small amount, as his intern's salary in the early 1950s was seventy-five dollars a month). In his penultimate entry, Rubin rejects the administration's request, presented by the offending Mr. Quistle, that he give a public interview after saving the life of a man on the street:

> Maybe the $1,000 is still burning me up, or maybe it's false modesty, or maybe it's that I feel it's inappropriate to fuss about something no one would think twice about if it had happened in the E.R. But whatever it was, I felt in my guts that for me no was a good answer, and it felt good to say it. He then congratulated me on being an excellent intern and said he was sure I'd be a very good psychologist. The s.o.b. doesn't even know the difference between a psychologist and a psychiatrist! (177)

The injustice of cultural discrimination in medical education and practice echoes throughout all the memoirs. Most often, the tension exists between physicians or students and their patients, but the dynamic of cultural difference applies to interprofessional relationships as well, as Rubin's experiences, including his own hostility toward Waggoner, demonstrate.

Of the five lengthy excerpts above, the third is the least focused. It is the one in which Rubin reports being exhausted after a twenty-four-hour shift. As he begins to describe the work, he realizes that in his first sentence he has written "eighty-eight cases." "Funny, me calling them cases!" he exclaims. "Just a few months ago I made big lectures to myself to remember that *people* must never become *cases* if I'm ever to become a decent psychiatrist when I leave here." Rubin's shock at hearing these pejorative words in his own voice is a familiar epiphany across the memoirs, and writers often use this unexpected, disappointing moment to reflect upon their development to such a point. After this interjection, though, Rubin resumes his reflection on how tired he is, how exhaustion stimulates his eating, and his worries about his weight. He seems to tie the bad hours to the world of nonpsychiatric medicine, or he may just be expressing his desire to be done with the rotation. He enters into a dialogue with himself about his mixed feelings about emergency medicine, then ends the entry with a vow to begin dieting. Rubin's concern about his weight, however, runs throughout the four months of his diary. In associating his struggles not to gain weight with the exhaustion and hard work he is subjected to (as in his complaint that it feels as if he saw "seventy of the eighty-eight" cases), Rubin implies that this workload is deliberately punishing him.

Two other aspects of this third excerpt draw my attention. The first is what has been called *embodiment*, which encompasses the writer's sense of being physically marked or changed by an experience, in this instance, Rubin's steadily increasing weight. The second, a concept closely related to embodiment, is vulnerability. Writers repeatedly express their fears of emotional and even physical exposure in an unsafe environment, in which patients can hate them or even die, teachers can harass or demean them, and their own bodies can tire or shed tears. In such overwrought situations, students and residents can feel anger or isolation. Rubin's concern about his weight not only involves his body in his daily experiences but also embodies his ongoing feelings of anxiety, frustration, and self-pity.

By the end of his four months in the E.R., intern Ted Rubin accepts, albeit unhappily, a dinner invitation from Kurt Waggoner. He meets and likes Waggoner's wife and daughters, and he grapples with feeling that it's "almost as easy to be forgiving" as it is to be hateful. "But it's a lot harder to feel it all at the same time," he concludes, "and that's how I feel—confused as hell" (176). He has saved the life of a man who collapsed on the street by using his medical skills. And he was given a hand-knit cashmere sweater by Logan, the hard-as-nails chief nurse of the E.R.: "I couldn't keep from crying, and Logan actually cried, too" (177). Although readers know, from presenter Rubin's introductory sections, that intern Rubin will eventually see these four months as crucial ones in the formation of his professional identity, readers have nevertheless been able to share his own doubts about the value of his experience as he ricochets repeatedly from dismay to indignation to despair to triumph to amazement, asking himself what he is to make of all this as a future psychiatrist and as, himself, a tender psyche. Emerging from his personal ponderings, however, are questions about power, relationships, and the embodied nature of medical practice that resonate throughout all of the memoirs of medical education.

Kenneth Klein, circa 1973–1977

Twenty years later, around the time that Rubin's son was undergoing his residency, Kenneth Klein was entering medical school. Although documenting an earlier phase of medical education, Klein records a similar process of gaining confidence over an incredibly short course of time. *Getting Better*, the book's jacket indicates, was published while Klein was specializing in gastroenterology at Oregon Health Sciences Center, which means that he probably wrote this book during his residency years, placing him less than five years past the last events he describes. Klein has not, to my knowledge, published any further memoirs, but he has accumulated an impressive list of publications in the biomedical sciences. He eventually moved into the pharmaceutical industry, designing clinical trials and coordinating the strategies for manufacturing, regulating, and marketing a number of drugs. In 1996, he founded Endpoint, which offers worldwide consulting in pharmaceutical development.[5]

Klein attended Harvard Medical School, which he names in his book. He does not indicate that he has changed any names in the telling of his experiences. (I mention this detail in the three memoirs I examine here, because there is growing concern about confidentiality and a writer's "ownership" of a story that involves other people's lives. The issue takes on an even greater import when patients have not been asked for permission to tell their stories.) Klein reproduces a diary of his third-year clerkship in internal medicine when he recounts those weeks, but all the other chapters are written retrospectively. The book unfolds chronologically except for the prologue, which describes an incident from the emergency room during Klein's third year. The frame is deliberate. Klein ends his book with a parallel situation at the end of his fourth year, and he uses this device to contrast the green third-year student with the budding confidence of the med-school graduate less than two years later. The book's title, no doubt deliberately ambiguous, can mean either that Klein is becoming more medically skilled or that he has grown better able to handle emotionally the challenges he faces.

Although there is no reason to believe that Klein would fabricate either of the two events described here, the following passages, one from the prologue and one from the last chapter, demonstrate how the author has connected the two experiences in his mind, seeing in them a detailed mirror of his technical and emotional growth:

The patient wore a flannel shirt, chinos, and a day-old beard. He lay on the steel stretcher, breathing regularly; from a distance he could have been sleeping. But when I put my hand on his shoulder to say hello there was no response. For a change I was spared the awkwardness of introducing myself as a medical student to a patient who was expecting a doctor. I picked up the emergency ward sheet that lay on his chest. His name was Richard Hastings. He was seventy-two. The triage nurse's note read: "Found unresponsive on bedroom floor. Period of unconsciousness unknown. Brought in via ambulance with diagnosis of stroke. Vital signs stable."

I started my exam with the patient's head. While working my way through his stringy hair I found a deep laceration on the right temple. Had he suddenly lost consciousness, then fallen, and hit his head? Or did he hit his head first, becoming unconscious because of the injury? I began a detailed neurological exam, looking for clues.

Mr. Hastings's breathing grew irregular. Also, his right pupil seemed to be getting bigger. His lungs and his eyes were telling me that a little lake of blood had formed beneath the skull and was beginning to compress the brain—Mr. Hastings had a subdural hematoma. To help confirm my diagnosis I tested the reflexes. Sure enough, there were no reflexes on the left but they were normal on the right. So the head injury came first! . . . It was glorious to see my studying at last beginning to pay off. Instead of merely reading a case history, I was seeing physiology in the flesh. I ran to the chief resident, Eric Costello, rejoicing over my unconscious patient.

Physiology continued to unfold before my eyes—just as we arrived back at Mr. Hastings's stretcher, he stopped breathing. Eric grabbed the laryngoscope and an endotracheal tube from the crash cart and called for help. Within seconds he had threaded the tube down the patient's windpipe. A nurse appeared and hooked up an Ambu bag; Eric began to squeeze it rhythmically, breathing for Mr. Hastings. For me this had been the transition from neuroanatomy to terror. But for Eric the intubation led as naturally from the patient's respiratory arrest as the respiratory arrest followed from the expanding clot of blood.

Doctors and nurses came running from everywhere. I was both thrilled and depressed at the incredible burst of activity. . . . How could I ever understand, much less hope to do, all that I saw going on? My pretty little piece of physiology had dissolved into a complicated mess.

A neurosurgeon appeared and even that depressed me—how did you get a neurosurgeon in an emergency? Eric quickly told him the story. I was astounded to hear Eric say, "It was this medical student Klein here who diagnosed the subdural." There was no basking in my fragile glory though: "Excellent," the neurosurgeon said. "Since my resident is sick, Dr. Klein can assist at surgery and actually see the clot he diagnosed."

I was terrified. My only real operating room experience had been removing the spleen from a black and white mongrel in dog surgery lab. . . .

[Alone with Mr. Hastings on the seemingly endless ride up the elevator to the operating room, Klein panics, as he struggles to keep "bagging" Mr. Hastings, squeezing air from an inflatable bag into the unconscious man's lungs.] I grew angry at Eric for handing Mr. Hastings over to me, then at the City of Boston for putting me in this situation by not hiring enough staff. Then the anger turned inward. I grew angry at myself for stupidly choosing the Boston City [Hospital] to do my emergency ward rotation. I grew angry at my incompetence, at my pretense at trying to play doctor, and at my decision to go to medical school in the first place. The elevator stopped at the seventh floor and I got out. . . .

[Mr. Hastings dies during surgery, and Klein's terror only deepens.] The only sound in the room after Rogers's last squeeze was the hissing of the respirator, still ventilating Mr. Hastings's lifeless lungs. Did I do this, I wondered, by improperly bagging him on my nightmare trip to the operating room? Am I the one who caused this surgeon to lose his first case?

Rogers suddenly severed the stillness. He took my hand and placed it on the warm rubbery heart. "Here, practice squeezing this," he said. "You might save someone's life someday." (3–5, 7, 13)

Klein begins his book in a tone that lightly mocks the green third-year student, thrilled to make a diagnosis that would be second nature to people skilled in emergency medicine. Delighted as the physiology he learned a little over a year ago has been confirmed in the flesh, he "rejoic[es] over [his] unconscious patient," a bit of ironic foreshadowing that warns the reader that Klein is no doubt headed for a fall. Which happens almost immediately, sending Klein from dizzy euphoria to dismay to panic to anger. His focus turns to his fear of his inability to properly don surgical garb, and his self-doubt continues to grow as Mr. Hastings dies on the operating table, an event that the surgery resident says has never happened to him before. Klein is left with the warmth of Mr. Hastings's newly silenced heart in his hand and the vague words (of solace? of blame?) of the resident ringing in his ears.

Less than two years later, Klein is driving to an interview for a residency in internal medicine in Burlington, Vermont, at Mary Fletcher Hospital. Outside a small town near Burlington, Klein comes upon a highway accident. He offers to stay with the injured man while another onlooker goes for help, although he feels "more like a voyeur than a physician." He continues,

> Suddenly I was alone with this man who seemed to be barely living. A seed of panic sprouted in my belly. I recognized that feeling well. It had been there on and off all through medical school. It was there that night in the emergency ward when Mr. Hastings had stopped breathing. . . . But at least I had been in the hospital. . . . Even so, Mr. Hastings had died.
>
> "Oh God. My leg, my leg," moaned the man.
>
> I put my hand on his shoulder. "Hello. My name is Ken Klein. I'm a medical student. You've been in a bad accident. Help is on the way."
>
> "My leg, God, my leg!" he chanted. . . .
>
> [Klein finds gasoline dripping from a punctured gas tank and fears for their safety, but he decides against moving the man.] So I was stuck with this injured man in his time-bomb truck, waiting for the ambulance. What could I do for him in the meantime? Think, I said to myself, think! . . .
>
> Again I thought of Mr. Hastings. There was blood caked onto this man's hair. What if *he* had a subdural? I took off his cap and surveyed his bloody head. The left ear was badly cut. It was slowly dripping blood. . . . I combed my fingers through his hair, feeling for fractures. But there weren't even any scalp lacerations; all the blood was from the ear. . . .
>
> [Klein describes the examination he is able to perform within the cramped seat of the car.] He lay against my chest; my arm supported him around the upper part of his back. It was nice to feel his body against mine; it made him feel more alive. (265–67)

Klein's introduction of himself to this man reflects his ongoing effort to present himself honestly to his patients, at a time when the usual practice was to refer to all medical students as "Doctor." His patient's condition immediately calls up memories of Mr. Hastings and triggers Klein's as-yet-unconquered feeling of panic in uncertain situations. His medical experience, however, holds him in good stead, as he quickly ascertains that this man has no fractures or lacerations on his head. The weight of the man's body against Klein's as they await the ambulance is reassuring, as it physically conveys a sense of the man's sentience, in stark contrast to the lifelessness of Mr. Hastings's heart in his hand.

The ambulance arrives and Klein follows as the paramedics take the man to a local emergency room, where they give the man, now identified as Mr. Shelton, enough treatment to move him safely to the better-equipped hospital in Burlington. Klein again follows the ambulance. The emergency ward at Mary Fletcher is as busy as the one at Boston City Hospital, but Klein is taken back to the room where Mr. Shelton is being treated. He is welcomed by the physicians treating Mr. Shelton and learns that one of the concerns he had expressed to the physician at the first hospital had led the physicians to discover that Mr. Shelton was bleeding into his abdomen. Klein is invited to watch the surgery that saves Mr. Shelton's life, which he does eagerly.

After the surgery, Klein leaves the hospital to spend the night with his friend Fred, who is an intern at Mary Fletcher. Over dinner with Fred and Harold, another intern, Fred recounts all he's learned in the past few months, and Klein muses, "Fred seemed so competent. Like Harold, he seemed much more mature than I, and obviously knew so much more. And like Harold, he was only twelve months ahead of me in his training. How could I ever hope to catch up to him?" (280). Klein answers his own question the next day, as he is being taken on a tour of the hospital:

> The tour passed by the intensive care unit. Among the anonymous row of the critically ill I saw a familiar face. I ducked out of the tour and went to his side. I stared at the quilted-together ear that had bled on my shirt, at the thick chalky cast which held the leg I'd untangled from between the pedals of the truck, and at the chest tube which still sucked the blood that wasn't there on Dr. Peters's x-ray. Mr. Shelton was still intubated from surgery, lying passively as the respirator took his breaths. A nurse came by to adjust his IV. I asked her how the patient was doing and she got the chart for me to read; I guess she assumed I was a doctor. After fiddling with the IV, she started to reposition him in bed. I put down the chart and slipped a hand under his back and his thigh, to help her. "Be gentle,"

I said; "he's someone special." Suddenly I understood how it was possible to be sustained through an internship. (281)

The gently mocking tone in the prologue's first paragraphs is completely gone here. Klein ignores the misunderstanding about his professional status, a symbolic acknowledgment that he now accepts this role, at least where Mr. Shelton is concerned. His words also mark a new realization. When he began his medical education, Klein had expected to pursue research in neurophysiology (19). Patient care had been a means to another end, an engaging means, but not something that Klein had imagined would become an end in itself. The student's words to the nurse at Mr. Shelton's bedside may sound a bit pompous, but Klein the author has chosen to end his story with the importance of the relationship between physician and patient.

Unlike *Emergency Room Diary*, in which the senior Rubin strives to stand apart from his assessment of intern Rubin's reactions and judgments, *Getting Better* shows the author Kenneth Klein manipulating chronology and selecting details that best highlight the aspects of his professional and emotional development that he deems most pertinent to the story his title suggests. He demonstrates his greater medical competence and emotional maturity (even when still frightened) in such carefully paralleled details as the presentation of himself to his patients, his comfort in offering medical observations to senior physicians, the personal embodiment of his connection to Mr. Shelton and his separateness from Mr. Hastings, and the different sense of responsibility and affection he felt toward these two men.

Whether these details of Klein's experiences registered thus with him at the time, they arose from his memory as he wrote, and the process of writing allowed him to demonstrate how he had changed by the way he chose to write his story. Klein thus uses literary artifice to recreate as pointedly as possible his emotional experiences. He could step out of his story to comment, as presenter Rubin does in his introductory sections, but narrator Klein has chosen to dramatize the changes in student Kenneth Klein without the gloss of a voice removed in time. Although his choice of details makes his assessment clear, he still allows his readers to reach their own conclusion. Yet he ends his memoir on a note of a new beginning that echoes the hope and spirit of the New World: "I had matched with my first choice, the program in Portland, Orgeon. I ran to the phone to call Phyllis. We were going west, to begin our new lives" (284). Go West, young man! Klein sets out for the frontier (as a good man of the mid twentieth century, with his woman at his side), freshly minted from his struggles to face and conquer whatever lies ahead.

Emily Baldwin, 2000–2002

Rubin and Klein both published diaries they kept for themselves during the years of their medical training. Emily Baldwin knew her diary would be read by strangers from the moment she entered a computer command that sent her words to the World Wide Web. Although public instead of private from its beginnings, the form of Baldwin's writing places her (and the other bloggers in my reading) in a different relationship to her story and her readers than exists for any of the other memoirists. Diarists write without knowledge of the future, even though they have some distance in time from the events they describe. Other published diaries that I cite here were written a few years or even a few decades before their authors chose to print them. Writers like Perri Klass, who was publishing essays while a student, went through a formal process that submitted their words to review and revision, undoubtedly by editors and the authors themselves. Thus, these online diaries possess an immediacy not present in diaries published in more traditional venues.

Emily Baldwin was one of eight medical students who were designated diarists—bloggers, in the world of the Internet—on medschooldiary.com, created in 2000 by cousins and first-year medical students Daniel Imler and Brian Hartman. The eight diarists included two women and six men, one man and one woman older than their classmates, one man of South Asian heritage, and two of the six in osteopathic medical schools (as opposed to the more numerous allopathic schools—DO the designation of graduates of the former, MD of the latter). In a short time it became the most widely read medical-student blog site internationally, and within a year or so became a part of a larger site, Student Doctor Network, a not-for-profit organization operated by the Coastal Research Group. Hartman and Imler created medschooldiary.com (and, after their graduation, its spinoff, residentdiary .com) for the express purpose of letting people contemplating medical school know "what it's like."[6] In addition to the diaries, each writer's site permits readers to respond directly to the diarists, who then post those responses at their discretion, sometimes with their own responses to the responders.

Another feature, not used by all the diarists, is a "quiz," in which diarists can pose a question with multiple choice answers for readers, with another link to view the tally for each response. Questions range from the technically medical to the personally whimsical, but they also offer another window onto the writers' thoughts and lives.[7]

The eight diarists of medschooldiary's earliest years are not by any means the only medicine-related bloggers (although this site is probably one of the most consciously structured and managed). These eight are also the ones most deliberately focused on writing about medical education. The full range of medical students and interns writing blogs today (the very term did not exist when Baldwin and her cohort began posting their diaries) echoes the breadth of writing within the phenomenon of the blog. Politics, travel, and samplings from other blogs and print media are as likely to be the object of these writers' attention as they are on anyone else's blogs. Medical students, residents, retired physicians, nurses, and nearly all other health professionals are represented. In short, health professionals write in every medium and genre electronically, as they have done in all other literary venues across the years. Blogging, as a mode of writing, has its own hallmarks and stylistic issues, which I shall consider when they are relevant to this study.

Emily Baldwin began writing for medschooldiary.com soon after her arrival at the University of California San Francisco (UCSF) School of Medicine in August 2000. Baldwin is a graduate of Swarthmore College and the Harvard Graduate School of Education. She taught high-school English and worked in a variety of jobs before beginning medical school. She expects that her age and background will, she tells her readers, make her "perspective . . . a little different . . . [but] I hope it makes for good reading."[8] Readers of her diary often compliment her on her graceful writing style, gentle humor, and compassionate descriptions of patients. Other readers, however, are put off by her entries. Extreme—and extremely expressed—responses from readers appear across all the diaries in medschooldiary.com and are common in the culture of blogging itself. All the bloggers have both ardent fans and equally ardent detractors.

Undergraduate medical education by 2000 had undergone changes since Rubin's and Klein's day, most noticeably in the amount of contact students have with patients in the first two years of medical school. Where Klein would have lecturers occasionally bring a patient into a lecture hall, Baldwin went regularly to talk to patients in the office of a local practitioner, got to know a pregnant woman who was being seen at the medical center, and spent time with a medical team that went to a homeless shelter. Physicians gave lectures not only about medical conditions but also about their own illnesses and their own experiences of grief. The curriculum at UCSF also included electives in the humanities—in which Baldwin regularly enrolled—one of which was a writing course taught by physician-writer Rachel Remen that invited students to explore their emotional responses to their experiences in medical school. These kinds of courses have become a staple of many medical schools (and will be discussed in my conclusion), with the belief that they will make students more at ease with patients and with themselves as caregivers when they enter their hospital-based training.

Even so, medical school is not easy, and Baldwin's readers share her fears and triumphs as she moves through the first two years. But we see the anxiety over an anatomy exam fade as she discovers she has escaped unharmed. We feel her grief when the young mother she came to know suddenly loses her baby to Sudden Infant Death Syndrome, but we also are among the first to learn of Baldwin's engagement and follow the hassles that planning a wedding can layer onto an already over-crowded life. Like all the bloggers, Baldwin tries to record both the good and the bad, but human nature can often skew that balance, as it can in printed memoirs just as easily. Numerous times during her first two years Baldwin will follow a previous day's critical posting with a moving story about a physician or patient to remind herself—and her readers—that this is what is important, this is why she chose to leave teaching and take her chances in medicine.

Readers have only a few entries of Baldwin's diary that deal with emergency room experiences, some from a short in-hospital preceptorship late in her second year (a short, observational experience in which students follow an assigned physician at work) and some early in her third year as part of her clinical clerkship in internal medicine. One entry from each of these experiences is excerpted below:

It's been a mind-numbing [second] year of (often tedious and repetitive) 9 to 5 lectures, with a multiple-choice exam in one subject or another every Monday morning. It's hard to keep caring so deeply when you're taking your 55th multiple choice test in two years. . . .

I am more worried by the hardening towards disease—and, by extension, towards patients. I have a preceptorship in the ER of SF General Hospital, and I've learned an enormous amount there about the presentations and complications of common illnesses. It's exhilarating, and yet I also notice that I am relating to these patients differently than I would have a year ago. Knowing more now about the features of, for example, diabetic ketoacidosis, I find myself focusing more on the right questions to ask, anticipating a particular answer, noting carefully when the presentation seems atypical in some way. . . . I am proud of this developing skill, since it's not an easy one. I am also worried. . . . Sometimes I find myself frustrated as I listen to a patient describe things that I already know are not going to be relevant to their "chief complaint." . . . And I don't even have the excuse of the intern—I am not so busy that I simply don't have time to listen to the details. I'm only a second year, I have nothing but time—but still I find myself hardening.

And, finally, there are the times—most difficult of all—when the hardening isn't enough. When I feel myself growing soft and fearful and upset in the face of some new medical horror. . . . Last night, for instance, I learned to suture. I was clumsy and slow, and completely clueless about sterile procedure (which no one had ever managed to explain to me before, but which felt like some kind of sadistic version of a kid's game. Like trying not to step on the cracks in a brick sidewalk). The intern was kind of frazzled as he'd instruct me in something basic—how to put on sterile gloves—but forget to mention some other detail. Every other sentence—No. Don't put your hand there. That's contaminated the field. Do it over. Keep your hands in close. Don't touch anything. Well, you can touch that. Your sleeve just touched the lidocaine bottle, it's contaminated. Hold this way. Don't move. Move. Do it again. Over. Another time.

My hands were shaking, I was painfully slow and cautious, but all the defenses in the world didn't stop me from thinking mostly about the patient. And maybe this was at least part of the basis of my problems.

She came in with big lacerations in her wrists (in the strange logic of the ER, these are apparently good training lacs for medical students, since they are straight and easy to sew). She was supposed to start her heroin detox program today, but instead decided to slit her wrists—and no wonder, really, that it would seem like an easier and less painful solution. When she woke up, she lay on the hospital bed and sobbed, long gasping breaths. I held her hand in my sterile glove, whispered softly, told her she was safe now, and tried to focus on my contaminating elbow and my 12 disobedient thumbs.

I couldn't sleep last night. I kept thinking about her lying there, in the harsh bright lights, sobbing convulsively and fearfully at the ceiling as the heroin started to gradually wear away.

As I left last night, she whispered up at me, "You're a nice nurse." I didn't bother to correct her impression. But I didn't feel like either one of the terms was especially true.[9]

The literature of medicine is filled with images of redemption and power. From "Learning to Play God" to "The House of God," [respectively, memoir and fiction by Robert Marion and Samuel Shem, both cited in this study] the implication is there: as physicians, we can make the choice to save lives or to let them go. With our knowledge and skills, we hold the power to heal and to cure.

Or so we would like to believe. . . . Here in the world of Inpatient Internal Medicine, however, where I am spending my first 8 week rotation, I believe that I am learning more of the grotesque, the absurd, and the pathos of humanity than I have learned of God.

After days that are anywhere from 12 to 20 hours long, with only four days off in the month, my mind is filled with stories that I haven't been able to fully process or understand. . . . Some of this haunts me in dreams: a plastic bedpan filled with cups of blood when an elderly man comes into the ED with an upper GI bleed. Night after night, lying in bed, I unwillingly remember helping the nurse to roll his enormous body, swollen with the ascites of liver disease, so that she can clean away the blood and shit from under him as he cries weakly, "Just let me die. I want to die." This is someone's grandfather, I think to myself. And when I see him the next day, after an emergency procedure has cured his bleeding and sleep has restored some of his dignity, I do not mention the terrors of the night before: he has forgotten the details, and I do not tell him that I saw him at his lowest moment. . . .

A woman my age is referred here from another hospital. I learn that she, like myself, was recently married. Not long after the wedding, she started having strange pains and nauseas, and thought joyfully that she was pregnant. She has just learned that there is no baby, but that the thing growing inside her is a malignant melanoma. She is unlikely to live longer than a year. Each morning when I see her on rounds, I am devastated once more by her face: her pale skin and dark hair framing huge eyes that look out at me, sad and tired and afraid. I feel guilty for my own joyful wedding, for the fact that I am standing at the bedside in a clean white coat, while she is lying in a tangle of tubes and flashing machines. . . .

And it doesn't end. The man who comes to the hospital thinking he has food poisoning, but who turns out to have a terminal liver cancer instead. . . . The elderly woman who cries in her room, whose daughter brought her to the hospital days ago, but who now refuses to come and pick her up. . . . The elderly woman who lived a completely independent life until she was hit by a bus and suffered cranial bleeding, and who now lies semi-comatose in her bed, punctuating the silence with odd fragments of some unintelligible, mournful Irish song.

I become less afraid of touching people's hands, of whispering to them in the chaos and bright lights of the Emergency Room. "It's going to be okay," I say quietly, and maybe I'm saying it for them, and maybe I'm saying it for me. Is this playing God? I can't imagine anything further from the truth. In fact, I can't think of any analogy, it is so different from anything I've ever done. But if I had to make a comparison, I'd say it was more like ministering, as I am brought each day face-to-face with the strangest and most terrifying realities that humanity can offer up. And in the face of it, we comfort, we offer the best we can, and, if we have anything to do with God at all, it is not because we emulate deities, but rather because we pray to them. We pray that there is another power out there that can heal these people, since it is so clear that the tools we have in our own grasp are painfully, absurdly inadequate.[10]

At thirty-two, Baldwin is the oldest of these three writers, but her extra years fail to mitigate the emotional force of her experiences. She wrote initially that she hoped her years as a teacher would serve both herself and her readers well, but at times she wonders if she has the drive and motivation she sees in her younger classmates. This self-doubt, however, plagues nearly all students, whatever their age or background. Like the other writers, she is impatient with aspects of her education, exhausted from long hours in the hospital, and often feels that she is at the mercy of other people in her environment. She anguishes over her patients' lives, and her dreams are haunted by graphic details of their physical conditions. There is nothing here that does not appear in other memoirs, although, as with all the others, Baldwin's voice is uniquely hers.

Missing in these two entries, however, is the humor that inflects much of her earlier writing. It is often directed at the surrealism of medical education (an essay about students carrying boxes of bones home on the BART), the usually pointless attempts at mastering the onslaught of information (students who take notes with at least three colors of pens), the awkwardness and intrusiveness of unskilled medical students (the student who faints while observing a medical procedure in a tense, overcrowded room in the E.R.).[11] Baldwin often laughs at herself, but she also creates for herself the position of teacher, older and perhaps a bit more realistic about her limitations. In these two passages, Baldwin continues to comment on her actions and reactions, but her tone becomes more somber, darker, while still maintaining the lyricism of most of her postings. She writes on May 2, 2002, of a "hardening" that is both detrimental and necessary, but she fears its development. She is unhappy to find herself growing annoyed with patients who impede her systematic interview, an echo of Rubin's discomfort when he finds himself referring to patients as cases. But she is also upset when "hardening isn't enough," or, perhaps more accurately, when she is unable to achieve an emotional distance that will allow her to do needed work "in the face of some new medical horror." Concerned with more than technical inexperience, Baldwin writes in her last entry about horror that "doesn't end," followed by a catalogue of people suffering not only from illness but from the sad circumstances of their lives, conditions that are also described by Rubin and Klein.

At times she registers her work with patients in terms of touch. Again on May 2, 2002, her statement "I held her hand in my sterile glove" underscores Baldwin's sense of invasion and uselessness much as does young Klein's reaction while squeezing the warm heart of a man whose death Klein feared he had caused. Baldwin places a latex glove between her patient's hand and her own, producing a sense of "sterility" that leads her to disavow both the qualities attributed to nurses and those of, more simply, a "nice" person. In less than three months, however, she comes to view "touching people's hands" as perhaps "offer[ing] the best we can" in light of the "painfully, absurdly inadequate" tools that medicine has to offer. Baldwin's final word about her work in an emergency room echoes the same epiphany experienced by Rubin and Klein—perhaps a recollection more than a revelation—that she is drawn to medicine and held there, whatever obstacles she encounters, by her desire to care for patients with her heart as well as with her head and hands. It is the patients who reminded Baldwin, Klein, and Rubin, across a span of fifty years, why they wanted to be physicians, and it is an affirmation they cherish every time it occurs.

For an unknown length of time after this posting, Baldwin attached comments from her readers, mostly ones offering her encouragement and praise. But no new postings from Baldwin appeared. The cessation of her postings upset a number of readers, some of whom also posted to other diarists in hopes of learning whether Emily was still in medical school. Readers received no answers, but a Google search of Baldwin's name reveals that she completed medical school and has gone on to a residency in psychiatry, also at UCSF.[12] She was featured in a story about UCSF's medical humanities program, of which she was a strong advocate.[13] (I did not know, at the time I selected Baldwin's postings for this chapter, that she had gone into psychiatry, but I decided to keep two eventual psychiatrists' memoirs in this chapter because diversity of writing format, gender, and historical time were more important to my analysis at this juncture.)

Even more than the other students and residents who have decided to make their experiences public, the contributors to medschooldiary.com have made a risky contract with their readers: to offer, in Brian Hartman's words, to tell "what it's like" before knowing what they themselves are getting into. I do not know why Baldwin stopped posting. Another blogger also stopped writing abruptly. Most others found themselves posting less frequently after the second year, although a few still posted into their residency years and beyond. Neither can I say whether writing a blog helped Baldwin to better understand her experience. On February 2, 2001, she wrote about observing a woman giving birth, concluding, "I am clearly still thinking through a lot of what I learned yesterday, but one thought is very clear: yet again, I am realizing that the most profound moments (or at least in my extremely brief medical career) are moments that have little to do with clinical intervention)."[14] To a reader who thanked her for this entry, Baldwin wrote a little more about the effects of keeping the diary: "Thanks for the comments—I have really been enjoying writing about medical school, since it helps me to think through some of the experiences I've been having. I often forget that other people are reading them, however, so it's nice to get a reminder!"[15] This statement may be a bit disingenuous, as she and the other bloggers also take time to reply to some of the people who write them. Nearly all of them also report having their diaries read by other students and even faculty. And, like Baldwin, they all report surprise that people are reading what they write. Such responses underscore the paradoxical nature of life writing as an act that is simultaneously public and private.

These three writers, whatever the form of their memoirs and whatever their narrative stance, have made deliberate decisions to be commentators on the process of becoming a physician. They engage their readers with varying degrees of directness, and each writes in a voice that is uniquely his or hers. That said, there is a remarkable consistency of concern expressed across the years and personalities of these writers. The stories they choose to tell have allowed me to identify three issues that challenge us to rethink the nature and practice of medical education. Accounts of exhaustion, anxiety about creeping weight gain, and the feel of a dead heart in one's hand or the weight of an injured man on one's shoulder underscore the truth that medical education is an *embodied* as much as an intellectual process, with every cell of one's being responding to the transformation into a physician. *Power* infuses all aspects of the student's or resident's work as well, whether it be a sense of powerlessness in the face of racial discrimination or at the hands of seemingly punitive superiors or a sense of power in the ability to diagnose a patient's injury or give orders to others about the care of a patient. *Relationships* with patients, even when patients are barely conscious that a bond is being formed, fill the minds and hearts of medical students and residents, and grappling with one's fears or grief regarding patients must take place at the same time that one is also struggling to establish comfortable working relationships with peers and colleagues.

And, running throughout these broader issues are more particular pressures. They include the pressure of managing overwhelming amounts of information, work, and emotions; gaining competence in the technical skills of medical practice, problem-solving, and what is often and rather insufficiently called communication skills; and developing a sense of one's personal as well as professional identity. These pressures will be heard in the quotations about the different phases of medical education outlined in chapter 2. The context of learning and the kinds of skills taught will change, but the pressure and subsequent anxiety will simply reshape itself to fit the new situation. Still, whatever their doubts, these three people hold to their belief, at times barely expressible, that this is what they want to be doing. In all the examples of the negative aspects of medical education that will follow (although I try to include the positive ones as well), the occasional despair or anger voiced by most of these writers, in effect, offers proof of their hopes for the promise of medicine and the humanity of its practitioners.

Water from a Fire Hose

MEDICAL EDUCATION IS a continual process of initiation and self-discovery. So, however, is life in general. Memoirs of medical education are also stories about growing up. Students bring values and beliefs, often unexamined, to the classroom and clinic, but their ongoing social and moral development will henceforth occur within the crucible of medicine. Most medical students are in their early to mid-twenties. Some have married but most are single. School has tended to be easy for them, and they are accustomed to being at the top of their class. In addition to pursuing a rigorous academic program, many of them have also participated in programs of research or service relevant to medicine and in extracurricular sports, music, and fraternal or religious groups. When they enter medical school, however, their worlds dramatically narrow. They soon find themselves almost exclusively in the company of other medical students, whose aptitudes and goals closely resemble their own. They confront human mortality in the flesh when, on the whole, they themselves feel in the bloom of health. And they encounter philosophical paradoxes and political injustices, abstract dilemmas made flesh in the suffering bodies of their patients, at a time when many of their own philosophical and political positions have not yet been fully articulated or tested.

At the same time that they are encountering an array of cultural and meta-physical challenges, medical students are struggling to master an overload of new information, skills, and relationships, all of which must somehow transform a young man or woman into Doctor, an identity shaped not only by their own expectations but also by the expectations of teachers, loved ones, and—most crucially—patients. A widely used simile likens medical school to trying to sip water from a fire hose. This image draws upon two elements that are nearly universal in medical education: the voluminous amount of information that students encounter and their sense of helplessness as they face that deluge. Learning to accept the impossibility of ever being able to drink fully or comfortably from that fire hose is a pragmatic, intellectual, and psychological process that engages these people throughout their years as medical students and residents. The following chapter sketches the particular challenges of each year of medical school, offering at the same time an overview of the medical curriculum, which has changed somewhat in form and substance, but little in impact, over the fifty-plus years spanned by these memoirs.

Undergraduate Medical Education

YEAR ONE   Most of the first two years of undergraduate medical education (UGME) is devoted to what are called the basic sciences: anatomy, physiology, biochemistry, microbiology, pharmacology, and pathology. (The advent of molecular sciences and the swiftly expanding knowledge of genetics has altered the emphasis or scope of some of these disciplines over the years.) In the first year, however, one course—gross anatomy—continues to be most associated with a student's entrance into the profession of medicine. Students continue to anticipate it with a range of emotions, from almost euphoric eagerness to deep dread. Many people have called it the student's introduction to death; others have called the cadaver the medical student's first patient.[1] The students themselves often struggle to understand their relationship to their cadaver. Philip Reilly describes slipping into the anatomy lab before the start of class:

> I held my breath and tiptoed to my table. I grasped one corner of the surprisingly heavy blanket and slowly pulled back until I could see flesh. A layer of thick, clear plastic lay underneath the outer shroud. Through it I could see what vaguely resembled a human leg. The shape was right, but the color was all wrong. . . . I dropped the blanket, backpedaled to the door, and retreated. Perhaps it was better to let my curiosity simmer for a few more days. (4)

Dan Imler's anticipation of gross anatomy contains unexpected second thoughts when a cadaver is brought into the lecture hall:

> It was weird because about half of our class leaned forward to get a better look because they were super interested and the other half leaned back in shock of seeing a dead body. It was interesting to see which kind of

personality did what. It honestly wasn't that obvious. Personally, I leaned forward.

It was kind of crazy though when the prof. pulled out the arm of the female cadaver and you could still see the fingernail polish on her hands. It really put me back into focus that this was a real person after all and not just an anatomical specimen. All of a sudden I found myself wondering who she had been, what she had done and who had loved her. It was hard to imagine that just a few years ago she was up and active as I am today. What a scary way to have your mortality thrown in your face. Death really does exist.[2]

Although some students are never at ease in gross anatomy, most of them come to terms with it in a variety of ways. Reilly, after his early swift departure from gross anatomy lab, comes to enjoy his long hours of work there, writing,

In the stillness of the deserted room, the bulk of the morning's dissection complete, I could savor the beauty of the body's parts. One snowy afternoon slipped away as I marveled at the muscles of the leg. . . . Touching the sartorius gave deeper meaning to Baryshnikov's dancing and the paintings of Degas.

Anatomy dissection was the first time I had ever really been required to work with my hands. The discovery that I was not a complete klutz had real therapeutic value. I even started to fantasize about becoming a surgeon! (14, 18–19)

Frank Huyler describes seeking temporary refuge when the work weighs too heavily on him:

Three weeks later we carried his leg to the sink and washed the green stool out of the attached portion of his rectum. For the first time, it was too much, and I had to step outside, onto the high balcony. It was hot and still, and I held the railing, looking out over the pine forests that stretched for miles into the distance at the edge of town, knowing that I should go back inside. But I stood there anyway, emptying myself, until someone opened the door behind me.

"Are you OK?"

"I'm all right, Tony, thanks. I'll be there in a minute." (13)

The taboos surrounding dissection make all writers aware that they have entered a realm forbidden to most people.

Although gross anatomy tends to consume the imagination and, at least at the start, much of the emotional energy of first-year students, this is only one course in a fast-paced year. Students entering medical school expect an onslaught of new words and facts; even so, they nearly all underestimate the amount of material they will be asked to absorb and parrot back. Charles LeBaron complains,

> So what I was so diligently studying, like a half-literal medieval scribe copying out the New Testament, barely reading or understanding it, did have scope, grandeur, even a terrifying beauty. . . .
>
> I knew the letter of biochemistry. But had I understood the spirit? Since it was a rare lecture that mentioned anything but the isozymes of rabbit muscle aldolase, I was on my own. (72)

And blogger Emily Baldwin wonders "what to take away from this unpleasant and exhausting experience. In part, I think I learned a lot about how to study for the next [test]. I know at the beginning of the semester I was taking the approach of 'getting the big picture' rather than memorizing details, which seems pretty laughable now."[3]

Students who start out with the best-laid study plans are soon behind in one or more subjects. This progression is most dramatically demonstrated in the online diaries, whose writers find time each day to mark a new high or low in their studying efficiency. Take, for example, the following sample of numerous such entries by Dan Imler:

> 8/23/2000 . . . . Thank goodness I honed my time management skills in college, otherwise I'd be up a creek. Let that be a warning to you premeds . . . [Imler's ellipsis]
>
> I'm starting to get a little scared about this first test.[4]

> 9/24/2000 . . . . Oh my gosh am I d[y]ing!!!! I can only take a second to write today, because I think that I'm going to have a nervous breakdown from studying so much. Honestly, I have never felt so unprepared for a test in my entire life! It's not that I haven't worked on it (50+ hours the last week), but that there is so much material. By the time you have gone through everything you forget what you started with.[5]

> 10/23/2000 . . . . I figured I [could] give a little insight into what it is like to study for a medical school test. . . . I have tried to study about 3 hours a night for the last 3 weeks and then about 6 hours a night for the

last week. For me the best way to study has been to take notes in class, add notes [from] the syllabus, which outlines everything, and then finally bring it together by reading textbooks. . . . By now I think that everyone has pretty much found their own study habits, but it has gotten difficult to start.[6]

2/11/2001 . . . . The next test is quickly approaching and I have done NOTHING to prepare for it. Oh well, it's a good thing that I got all that experience cramming in college, it should pay off now![7]

As many of these postings indicate, complaints about large amounts of material to study usually accompany anxiety about exams.

The demands of study quickly begin to take their toll. Symptoms of sleep deprivation appear within the first few weeks, as reported, respectively, by bloggers Brian Hartman and Emily Baldwin:

What a nice day of relaxation. I skipped anatomy lab so I could come home and take a well needed nap. I crashed around 4:30 and woke up at 7:15. Now it's 2 AM and I can't sleep. Ugh.[8]

I didn't sleep so well last night, since I kept waking up thinking about the phrenic nerve and what the points of attachment are for the pectoralis minor. Ah, Anatomy. As a result, I was having a harder time today than I usually would.[9]

Students describe the psychological toll of always feeling behind. Perri Klass characterizes herself thus: "I am not easy to live with this year. I am always worrying about one test or another, I am always talking about things that don't mean much to non-medical students . . . and, most of all, I am very busy. And I am more than a little self-righteous about my busyness. Of course I can't do the shopping, I'm a medical student. Of course I can't wash the dishes, I have studying to do."[10] Often at some point in the second semester, students become acutely aware of despondency or depression, even though, as in Brian Hartman's blog, they never specifically identify it as such:

For some reason I've not been in the mood for medical school lately. I mean it started about a month ago. We had those two weeks of tests that killed me and then I got sick for a week before spring break. Now the week after break and I still can't seem to be able to study for more than a few hours at a time. I get easily distracted and spend lots of time researching stuff online about fish [he's recently bought a fish tank] instead of doing what I should be. Maybe if I start working out again I'll get the desire back. I defin[i]tely need something though because Monday I need to hunker down before the biochem and micro tests start looming on the horizon.[11]

There is a frequently voiced sense of loss, not just of time for exercise, music, or reading, but of connections with family and friends, as alluded to in Klass's words. Married students suddenly must ration their time with partners and children, a distressing circumstance even when others are supportive and accommodating. Dorothy Greenbaum's life changed so quickly that old habits vanished before she realized it:

That evening I curled up beside Eddie on the old familiar couch. As we sat side by side, I released an enormous sigh. This was the first night in ten months that there would be no barriers between us—no anatomy, no physiology or biochemistry, and no earphones [which Eddie wore so as not to distract Dorothy with his music]. Just the two of us. But Eddie was still on automatic. He slung his arm around my shoulders and put on his headset. I was too weary to object. I just began to cry. Midway through the song, Eddie turned and saw me, with my bloodshot eyes, crying silently. He took off the earphones.

"This is our first night together without the books. How can you do this?" I cried.

"Dorothy, I forgot. I honestly forgot." (129)

Mark Lee asked his wife, Angie, to write in his blog about her experience as the wife of a medical student early in the second semester of his first year. She begins, "Most of the time, Mark's being away doesn't bother me much. During the week, it's a lot like it was when he had a real paying job." But the tone changes as she describes her situation that weekend, alone with their three young children, one of them with a severe seizure disorder and developmental disabilities. "I also needed to pick up some photos and go to the grocery store. Mark is out of drinks and he can't study without his Diet Coke. Where is he when I need him? I didn't get that done, but I did cook one of his favorite meals—pork chops—for dinner. He will be home soon, and I'll have my family together."[12]

During the first year of medical school, students begin to take on a new identity. Although it is an identity they desire, for most of them it comes with consequences they had not anticipated: the shock of opening another person's body; the debilitation of sleep deprivation; the uncertainty of one's mental capacity to absorb vast amounts of scientific knowledge; the poignant distancing from close friends and family. And, although most students feel triumphant upon the successful completion of their first year and more confident in their ability to handle the information and pressures still to come, they express a range of assessments of the process they have just endured. "But I was learning medicine," Steve Horowitz says succinctly, his "but" encompassing all he must endure to achieve his goal (51). Dan Imler writes,

> I've had the hardest time coming down after the rush of tests and really this entire year. . . . I always wondered why my dad could never settle down until like the third day of vacation and now I know [Imler's father is a physician]. It's almost unsettling to be able to get up whenever you want to and have nothing hanging over your head. . . .
>
> I s[a]t back and reflected a lot this week about what this year has meant to me. . . . Probably the most important thing that I learned, personally, was a confidence in my own ability to succeed in med school. At the beginning of the year, you are afraid that perhaps you don't have what it takes to make it, perhaps college and the MCAT [Medical College Admissions Test] were flukes and now you sit with a 4.0 Harvard graduate with 39 MCATs and you have to compete. How the heck are you supposed to do that? The fact is, you just do. Whatever it is inside of you that motivates you kicks in and gets the crap done. As long as you came for the right reasons, you make it.[13]

Other students, such as Perri Klass, are less comfortable with their achievement. She wonders

> why I and many other people I know came here [to Harvard for medical school]: we want to be able to do what we want. I want to be a doctor who fits my own definition of a good doctor, and if that conflicts with other doctors' ideas, well, I want to have such impeccable credentials that they will still have to take me seriously. But the question is, by the time I finish, will I still remember any of what I originally wanted to be? When I am through with my training, will I have any way of knowing what kind of doctor I have actually become?[14]

In general, though, the students' moods upon completing—surviving, most of them consider it—their first year, are ones of jubilation, albeit sometimes cautious.

YEAR TWO   In the first year of medical education, the emphasis in the basic sciences is generally on "normal" body structures and functions. In the second year, students turn their attention to the "pathological" body, how structures and processes can go awry and lead to illness. (This distinction, between the perceived normal and abnormal is, itself, a powerful socialization in how most students will come to regard chronic illness, disability, aging, sexuality, and even pregnancy.) For many students, the amount of course-work seems more manageable, at least at first, as they are more familiar with the rhythms of classes and exams. Soon, however, the pace accelerates, and frustration and exhaustion mount once more. Students usually revert to their previous year's study patterns, but many of them respond with a cynicism that was lacking the year before, as do bloggers Ron Maggiore and Emily Baldwin, respectively:

> Well, now that I am skipping pharmacology right now and don't want to start reviewing my notes in the study lounge, I thought now would be a good time to post an entry. ;-)[15]

> A lot of people were talking today about how hard our respiratory exam was, and I suppose that's probably true, but I wasn't too concerned about it for some reason. I just didn't go in expecting to do great, so I guess I wasn't too surprised or something. Maybe low expectations can be a good thing sometimes. Maybe after all of these tests I am finally learning that it just isn't worth it to freak out about these things.[16]

To some extent these changes in attitude are a more reasonable approach to the amount of material the students face. Even so, their comments are often inflected with a sense of bemusement about their decreased desire to excel.

Money is a worry for many medical students (and residents as well). Because most medical students are expected to incur substantial debt, this is a secondary source of stress, but its constant presence adds to students' sense of insecurity. Ron Maggiore is not alone when he bemoans the mounting cost of books and equipment: "The final part [of M2 orientation] was essentials of clinical medicine, our physical diagnosis course . . . this threw everyone for a loop . . . three required texts and required medical equipment that is going to drain my savings . . . otoscope, ophthalmoscope, hammers and tuning forks . . . [Maggiore's ellipses] thank God I already have a stethoscope!! :-)."[17] Some students earn extra money by taking notes, part of a system in nearly every medical school that produces a detailed record of all the lectures, for which students pay a modest sum. Some students work while they are medical students, which most schools allow, cautiously, after the first year. Brian Hartman, who eventually worked in emergency rooms in local hospitals to augment his income, also seeks other sources of money:

> On a different note, I think I'm going to donate bone marrow for research. One of our professor[s] is a Heme/Onc guy who does research and they pay $100 per donation. You can do it every month. So I'm going to do that and transcribe notes [of class lectures] again next semester to get a little bit more spending money. Yay! The good thing is they take so little marrow it won't affect my blood donation schedule.[18]

In short, finances are often low-grade static in the background of medical education and residency.

Offsetting students' complaints about lectures and exams, the second year brings the welcome presence of patients. Over the past twenty years or so, medical schools have begun including what is called patient contact into the preclinical years. Although patient contact often begins in the first year, it occurs more extensively in the second. The earliest interactions usually take the form of simply talking to patients without performing any medical procedures. Sometimes students listen as physicians interview patients or as patients are brought into a lecture hall to talk about their medical condition. In Kenneth Klein's first class as a medical student, a physician brought an elderly woman into the lecture hall to illustrate his lecture on cardiac pacemakers. "I was astounded," Klein remembers. "This woman was perfectly willing to expose her chest in front of 140 total strangers. Somehow, because we intended to become doctors we were entitled to expect her to remove her blouse. How scandalous it would have been had she done the same thing in my chemistry class the year before!" (29). Dan Imler is amazed at the physician's power to explore taboo subjects with patients: "It was super interesting to have your first real patient interview experience. . . . I had never really dissected a person's background and honestly you have a power just by being a doctor that people think that they can tell you anything no matter how embarrassing or painful. It's quite amazing actually."[19]

As they begin talking to patients, students encounter one of their first ethical dilemmas: how to introduce themselves. In earlier years, there was only one approach. "In the spring quarter of the second year," writes Fitzhugh Mullan, "we were sent onto the hospital floors for the first time to see patients, as part of a Physical Diagnosis course. Indeed, it was the first time we examined living people with our own hands, the first time we were called 'Doctor,' and, perhaps most important, the first time we wore our white coats."[20] If the patients were fooled, however, no one else was. On one of her first visits to a hospital floor, Elizabeth Morgan remembers, "The ward secretary asked Dr. Vincenzo if we were new residents of his. He smiled and said we were joining him for rounds, which made us feel like real doctors until a resident looked up and said, 'That means they're first-year medical students'" (30). More recently, students and faculty are not quite as glib with premature titles. Today, many medical students introduce themselves as student doctor and give explanations similar to that offered by Stephen A. Hoffmann:

> Like most medical students, I was tempted to introduce myself as a physician. I feared that by acknowledging my status as a trainee I would risk rejection. The patient might refuse to allow me to take a history or to examine him (which would threaten my need to learn) or might be reluctant to trust and confide in me (which would threaten my sense of pride). . . . But however much I flirted with the idea of misrepresenting myself, I knew that a relationship based on deception wasn't possible. (122–23)

Along with talking to patients, most students in their second year begin touching patients. Some medical schools have students first practice the skills of physical diagnosis on other students. Although this does give students an appreciation of the vulnerability of the patient, it may also be dissipated by the awkwardness of appearing nearly naked among one's peers, a personal discomfort among friends that may not equate in their minds with the more unequal physician-patient relationship. Dan Imler reports skipping parts of the physical exam when the "patient" is another student: "It was the first time that we had to do the physical exam on a wom[a]n. My partner and I skipped several, shall we say 'personal,' exams to save our embarrassment. Oh well I guess it will get shot anyways next year when we have to do pelvic and rectal exams on real patients. I can't wait (sarcastic)!"[21] The stakes rise considerably, however, when it comes time to perform the same procedure on a patient. Issues of self-presentation again come into play as students wonder whether to reveal their inexperience to patients. In general, writers who report choosing to admit their inexperience feel better about the process in the long run. For example, from, respectively, Stephen A. Hoffmann and Perri Klass,

> To my surprise, I discovered that patients were not only remarkably receptive to having me participate in their care, but also remarkably forbearing.

I will never forget, for example, how graciously one woman put up with my efforts to place an intravenous line. As I tried repeatedly but in vain to enter a vessel, she astonished me with her patience, and when I told her, after several failed attempts, that I would find someone more experienced to do the job, she would have none of it, treating me to words of encouragement instead. Eventually I succeeded in getting a line in the poor woman, and when one of my residents happened to pass by, the woman commented with complete aplomb on how expertly I had inserted the needle. I could have kissed her. (122–23)

By now, reasonably sure that I can find the vein if it's there to be found, I am much less afraid to let the patient see if I am puzzled or unsure. "This will hurt a little, but I'll do it as quickly as I can," I say. Perhaps there is an implicit apology in my attitude, and that does not seem to me to be such a bad thing, because surely there ought to be some acknowledgment in such a situation that however necessary the pain may be, I am not the one who has to bear it.[22]

By the end of their second year, most students are more than willing to leave the lecture halls behind. They face one last hurdle: commonly referred to as Boards, it is the first part of a three-part national exam, the United States Medical Licensure Examination. Many medical schools require that students pass the first two parts in order to graduate from medical school. Part 1 covers all areas of the basic sciences that students have studied for the past two years; part 2 covers clinical knowledge and skills pertinent to the completion of undergraduate medical education and permits credentialing sufficient for the work of a resident. Part 3, taken at some point in one's residency, grants full eligibility for state licensure.[23] With their eyes now fully on clinical medicine, students often view the exam as a final insult or an irrelevance that nevertheless carries great consequences. Emily Baldwin captures the surrealistic roller-coaster experience reported by most writers:

And . . . it's over!
    After all the build-up, all the stress, and one long day of answering multiple choice questions, the USMLE is now one more item checked-off on my "to do" list. . . .
    So that's the USMLE. Frustrating, hard to predict, not quite the triumphant experience I had hoped for, but more a puzzling experience. Walked out of it kind of scratching my head and thinking, "Hmmmm.

Was that a dream?" But the main point is—it's over. And I finished it, and given that apparently most people pass, the odds are in my favor there. And yesterday it just washed over me, as I walked in the beautiful San Francisco sunshine and went out for a great dinner with my sweetie—I'm getting married in a little over a week! . . . I am tired today, and have a little post-exam stress headache, and I am also absolutely and deliriously happy.[24] (First ellipsis is Baldwin's)

Passing Boards is both a relief and an anticlimax. Life that was held at bay—often through most of two years—is finally allowed into the students' consciousness. Its beauty is often overwhelming.

YEAR THREE "Beyond the merest week break, the great unknown of third year loomed," Audrey Young writes of that almost imperceptible pause between lecture hall and hospital floor (44). The third year brings a dramatic change of venue and responsibility. Most students embrace it eagerly, whatever their nervousness. During their third year they rotate through five or six required clinical clerkships, each lasting from four to twelve weeks: internal medicine, pediatrics, surgery, obstetrics and gynecology, psychiatry, and (in most medical schools) family or ambulatory medicine. The majority of the work takes place on the hospital floors, although efforts have been made to increase the amount of outpatient or ambulatory work to better represent the patients a physician will most likely see in practice.[25] Students are finally in daily contact with patients, physicians, and other health professionals. Anthropologist Melvin Konner devotes most of his memoir to the third year of medical school because he felt it to be "the year in which the most important phase of socialization is largely completed, when the adoption of the values of physicians is effected. If at the end the acolyte cannot yet quite act or think like a physician, he or she can and does make moral judgments like a physician or, to be more precise (and this distinction will be important), like a house officer—a hospital resident or intern" (xiii). Immersed in the moment-to-moment experience, Jamie Taweel paints a more visceral picture of this liminal state:

Rotations have been a love/hate relationship thus far. To me, finally being in the hospital finally being able to deal with people, finally being able to put a face to those diseases I've been reading about—it's all worth it to me. I love it. I love working with the doctors. I love thinking that I'm going to soon be one of those doctors. I love talking to the patient. My big mouth finally pays off for once! . . .

Now for the hate: I hate getting pimped [a pseudo-Socratic method of questioning students that is often designed more to make students painfully aware of what they don't know than to teach them what they need to know—more about this later] into the ground with questions I don't know the answer to. I hate not knowing what to say or do. I hate it when a patient has a question I can't answer, and I have to tell them that. I hate stumbling over the diseases I know and not being able to pull the correct ones out of my head. . . . I hate the time I desterilized some equipment and held off the surgery until everything was replaced. I hate that I can't sincerely schmooze with doctors. They all have inside jokes that I wasn't around for.[26]

Often impatient with their inexperience and frustrated by their ineptness, students nevertheless find this a thrilling time.

The hospital itself is a confusing place, with warrens of hallways and an underground maze of labs and storage; in addition, students must regularly learn a new geography, as most medical schools teach in a number of hospitals. Each new rotation, moreover, contains a different cast of characters, similar only in their strict hierarchy: third-year clerks, then senior medical students; next, first-, second-, third-, and even fourth- or fifth-year residents; perhaps a fellow; and, at the pinnacle, the "attending," the only faculty person, who heads the "service" staffed by this "team." The attending is the person ultimately responsible for the student's grade but is probably the person least present during the student's long days on service.

Discomfort with learning procedures on patients continues, now magnified because of the greater number of tasks students must perform. The terror of drawing blood soon becomes mere annoyance, one of the many neverending assignments of "scut," chores that fill students' time with tasks that seem to keep them from more important (and usually more exciting) work they might be doing. Whatever other purpose it may serve, scut underscores the hierarchical nature of medical education. "Shit rolls downhill," a resident observes to student Elizabeth Morgan, as he heads home for the night. "Scut work is shit and we get it all. Good night" (49). Nevertheless, most students remain acutely aware of their inexperience. For a procedure to advance (or devolve) to the level of scut also signifies that the student feels some sense of mastery of that task and is eager for greater responsibility.

More problematic for third-year students are the distressing circumstances that often confront them. Death is clearly the most difficult of these. Most third-year students have never been with a dying person. Philip Reilly writes, "The first week of my medical clerkship was one of the most extraordinary of my life. It was the week that I became *familiar* with death" (111). Mark Lee describes his distress with his own impotence and the seeming nonchalance of a fourth-year medical student during a night on call in internal medicine:

> As M3s, my buddy Shane and I were taking orders from our team for supper from a local establishment . . . when the dreaded call came [from one of the floors, where a patient's heart had stopped beating]. . . . Everything was crazy. . . . The M4 on our team backed out of the room with Shane and me. He was a whiz kid type. Very smart and impressive. It was hard to believe that he was only one year ahead of us in his training. He looked over the scene glumly and remarked, "I haven't ever been to a code outside of the unit (ICU) that wasn't just a cluster f@*#." It was looking pretty clear that we were losing and our patient was not coming back. As our senior resident formally called a close to operations, our cool M4 turned to me and pulled a $10 out of his wallet. "I'll take the chicken strip dinner with fries and a coke." And with that the guy was declared dead, and the adrenalin rush was over. People began trickling out of the room. The family was escorted to the waiting room to share the bad news with the rest of the clan. The naked dead man on the bed looked violated with the line coming out of his groin and the endotracheal tube jutting from his mouth like some weird pacifier. Because he had a lot of gold jewelry on, Shane and I were given the first job of the night that I felt competent to handle. We were posted out in the hallway with instructions to let no [one] go in without authorization until the morgue could arrive. We only had to wait a short time before we were released from duty and headed out to pick up supper.[27]

Besides encountering death in their patients, many third-year students struggle to place these deaths into a larger cosmology that makes sense to them. Kenneth Klein, for example, writes in his diary toward the end of his medicine clerkship, "I feel strength in being able to see these deaths not as terrible tragedies, but as simply what must happen to us all. There is no dulling of feeling, but rather a sad resignation to what must be. I rejoice at being able to look at death so evenly, at being able to give some comfort to patients and their families. We will all die" (189–90). Philip Reilly responds to his sense of loss by taking intellectual action: "My first patient had died within hours after I met him. I simply could not believe it. Suddenly, a new duty loomed up.

My job was to learn clinical medicine, and in this business your patients were your professors. Mr. Webster still had something to teach me; it was my job to attend his autopsy" (113). Some students make a more private gesture, as does Stephen A. Hoffmann, whose patient died shortly after he had been given a test tube of the man's blood to take to the lab: "There was also the issue of what to do with his blood. Throwing it away was out of the question. Instead, I placed the tube in one of the pockets of my white coat and held it there for almost a week. It was the only substitute for a memorial I could devise" (183).

Exhilaration runs high, though, through the third year, often in the face of sleep deprivation. Now, students lose sleep not from studying for another in the interminable march of exams but from working late hours in the hospital. Being on call is a hardship that many students revel in as the surest mark of having arrived, as attested to by Steve Horowitz and Elizabeth Morgan:

Even with Dr. Walsh, I was being exposed to medicine, real medicine. And very real doctors. For the first time it wasn't books, advisors, plans. I was in hospitals, with patients, not just diagrams. I could at last make the connection between what I was doing and what I wanted to be. I was starting to feel like a doctor. (84)

That was Friday night. I was awake until Monday night, when I went home to sleep for the first time in sixty hours. For some reason, although I felt ignorant and did things wrong, I was having a wonderful time. (49–50)

But the long hours take their toll and lose some of their glamour as the year stretches on. A lot depends, also, on how much the student finds he or she enjoys either that particular specialty or the service's team. Ron Maggiore adds an emoticon of a winking eye to assure his readers that he is only joking about resorting to drugs after a long, late-night surgery: "Almost 2 weeks done with OB/Gyn. I'm post-call (second time around), w/ only 4 hours of sleep and am feeling like crap again . . . how am I supposed to read tonight for tomorrow's lectures?!? I really need some crystal meth to keep me going . . . ;-)" (Maggiore's ellipses).[28] John MacNab reports learning how to hold his own in giving a case presentation (the standard report on a patient's condition) to a particularly officious attending: "This last bit of mischief [was an outrageous, obviously bogus claim that] went right by the attending, who began to discourse on the recurrent nature of this disease. I was playing to the gallery, though, and the interns were choking with glee. Afterward I was praised for 'meeting pomposity with pomposity'" (192).

The third year of undergraduate medical education is a roller coaster of tragedy and comedy, of manic emergency amid tedious routine. Most writers take little or no pause to note the end of the year. Bloggers, whose posts often dwindle to one a month or even less during this year, register busy lives that are sweeping them along at a pace that allows little time to reflect or to connect with others. Ron Maggiore reports on an antici-pated evening in Chinatown with classmates, "Well, 3 of us showed up for karaoke but no one else did and the place never opened . . . [Maggiore's ellipsis] there goes my chance of singing 'If You Could Read My Mind' by Gordon Lightfoot! ;-)".[29] Dan Imler spends more time talking about his week's vacation with his family than he does the end of his clerkships: "So the end of my 3rd year of medical school has come and gone. Hey, and I'm still around to talk about [it], I guess this medical school stuff might not be so bad after all!"[30]

Imler's casual remark, however, implies hours when his mood was less rosy. Reflections from writers looking back from a greater distance run the gamut from delight to disillusionment, but all of them share recognition of the hard emotional work the third year involved. John MacNab captures the paradox inherent in much of medical education when he writes at the end of his third-year diary, "One of the important questions about the third year is why have I put up with it. The easiest answer is that it gets me into fourth year." A few pages later in an "Off-service Note," though, he explains to his readers why he has changed all the names in this diary, including his own: "I want to protect my medical school, which accepted me on a bet and has worked hard to teach me something. I am grateful. . . . But most of all, I want to be a doctor" (219, 222). For most writers, the desire to become a physician, whatever doubts they may have about their own abilities, has not changed. If anything, the year of constant interaction with patients has only reaffirmed that goal.

FOURTH YEAR   Many of the issues that confronted third-year medical stu-dents carry over into their fourth year, but the relief of having survived brings students to that year with greater confidence and a lighter spirit. Students scramble to take elective courses that will, they hope, support their residency applications or help them decide which specialty they want to pursue. They often revel in the technical language that has become comfortable in their mouths. Brian Hartman regales his readers:

Getting calls from nurses on diabetics and CHF patients is never a good thing.

I head up there and his glucose i[s] a solid 44. Appar[e]ntly the ER nurses didn't notice he didn't eat dinner and gave him 8 units of regular insulin from the SSI, and then 25 minutes later gave him the 10U of 70/30 he was supposed to get. Nice. Anyway, a few crackers, a pepsi, OJ, and an apple later his glucose was a solid 33. Crap. My interns were busy doing other things so I took the bull by the horns and ordered the first amp of D50 of my budding career. He was grossly diaphoretic and exhibiting mental status changes. To top it off, they also held his Lasix dose for the evening, so he was really fluid overloaded as well and satting 91% on 2L NC. Earlier his PO2 had been 58 while satting 95% so he was not correlating at all.

We had to have the meds sent up for him from the ER (again, they were sure trying to hurt me by not having sent them already). I then ordered Lasix 80mg IVP and waited for the fireworks, or the rain shower, depending how you look at it. Unfortunately, the shower came in the form of profuse vomiting all over the floor and I got to witness regurged pepsi, apples, OJ, and applesauce. Then just for kicks he lost bowel function and threw some stool around the bed. At this point my sphincter was a little tight and I too was developing a little diaphoresis. I mean he wasn't diuresing like I wanted. He was puking. He was hypoxic and hypoglycemic. The ward nurses were overwhelmed and all four nurses from the entire floor were there assisting.[31]

The post continues in this manner for four more paragraphs, eventually concluding, "Bottom line through all this was, I got to do most everything myself through all this, and learned a ton. There was one of my interns who hung around to help if I needed it, but for the most part I was OK. I finally felt like a doctor on this rotation and it made me feel great." Whether online or on paper, writers glorying in the mastery of medical detail seldom stop to explain the terms to their uninitiated readers. For all his insider bravado, however, Hartman's thrill with handling responsibility, albeit carefully supervised, rings throughout these lines.

Although students during their fourth year become more knowledgeable about the mechanisms of their patients' illnesses, they often become more frustrated about the course of those illnesses. In particular, they become upset with patients whose health might have been affected by their personal practices. Audrey Young writes about an unmarried, pregnant teenager:

> I left the room frustrated by the exchange. I couldn't understand why Amanda cared about her baby catching a rare disease when she poisoned her baby every day with carbon monoxide from cigarettes. In the free clinic, I'd met pregnant girls with similar histories whose previous children had been commandeered by the state and legal guardianship awarded to a distant relative. I did not often feel sympathy for these patients and I wondered if Amanda would face the same fate. (71)

Patients who do not want to do what the physician wants them to do can make students angry. Ellen Lerner Rothman writes about one such patient,

> I felt so frustrated and angry every time we argued with Roger, every time he refused another treatment. I knew he feared the drugs. I knew he tried to control his diabetes the only way he knew. More important, I knew he was frustrated with his situation. . . . We got so used to arguing with him that it became too easy to fight with him out of habit. He wasn't a likable person, and the residents and I found it hard to listen to him. . . .
>
> I knew I wasn't the perfect caregiver I so wanted to be. (152–53)

Some students struggle with these judgments; others draw on their growing sense of medical authority to support their indignation.

Besides gaining clinical self-assurance, a major activity of the senior year of undergraduate medical education is applying and interviewing for one's residency. Much of the students' talk in the fourth year trades in fact and rumor about different programs, various strategies for planning one's interview schedule, and a constant reshuffling of residency choices. The blogs often contain lengthy discussions of the pros and cons of the specialties and programs they are considering.

The last weeks of medical school offer another opportunity to take stock, to look back as well as forward, as do Ellen Lerner Rothman and Dan Imler below:

> After four years, my white coat finally feels familiar on my shoulders. Now grayed with use, one of the pockets has torn and is secured with staples as a temporary measure. I have grown accustomed to the rhythm of life in the hospital. Once awed by the medical intricacies depicted on *ER*, I now readily pick out the inaccuracies. Do I feel like a doctor yet? I'm still

not sure. I suspect I will never finish growing into my role as doctor and caregiver. (335)

So what does it mean to me now to be a doctor? Not much yet as all I've done with my degree so far is sleep in till 10am and occasionally tease my brother that he is still a mere mortal stuck in his 3rd year of medical school. But truthfully, the degree changes very, very, very little. I am still just as incompetent as I was before, I just have a greater probability [for] those weaknesses to cause problem[s]. I've tried to not let the pride of the title [a]ffect me too much.[32]

Kenneth Klein relates a more complex anecdote that marked for him the ways in which he had changed in just two years:

Already I'd forgotten how hard it had been at first; I was startled to learn how quickly death becomes routine. I sat with Ann [a third-year student] for a long time. I cried too, almost.

I told her she should come to Mr. Dugan's autopsy. Like intubating Krantz the night he died, going to Mr. Dugan's autopsy was unpleasant yet important. "It won't be easy," I said, "but I think you should go."

Ann and I talked afterward in the sweet and sour atmosphere of the morgue. She was shaken. She hadn't yet learned to pretend that seeing a dead person wasn't troubling. And not only was this her first autopsy, the body belonged to someone she had known, someone whose death it was now impossible to deny. . . .

So we talked and we learned from each other. From me Ann learned to push herself to get as much as possible from each medical experience. And from her I learned how much I'd changed since I'd been a second-year student. (252–53)

Klein describes his maturation in terms of both gains and losses—but losses that he is trying to remain aware of. For all the graduating students' sense of achievement, they know they are, once again, at the threshold of another beginning.

Graduate Medical Education

INTERNSHIP   Residencies begin, nationwide, on July 1. It is a standard joke (or aphorism) that a person does not want to be hospitalized in July, when medical students are suddenly physicians, junior residents suddenly senior. In short, everyone is usually unequipped psychologically for the new job title and lacks the year's experience of the interns and senior residents of the day before. Whereas most memoirs of undergraduate medical education begin with enthusiasm, sometimes laced with anxiety, most memoirs of residency begin with enthusiasm laced with abject terror, as Emily Transue and Michael J. Collins record:

> *This is Dr. Transue.* I stare dumbly at the attending for a moment, mesmerized by his words. I've waited for this for so long, worked for it for so many years. But now that it's happening, I'm not sure whether to be thrilled or terrified. (7)

> And misery it was. In less than twenty-four hours I had gone from the euphoria of beginning my career as an orthopedic resident at the Mayo Clinic to the feeling I was a counterfeit, an imposter who had infiltrated this society of brilliant surgeons. Once my ignorance was discovered . . . Dr. Burke would emerge from the shadows [of his office] and tell me a mistake had been made, a terrible mistake. (7–8)

In reality, first-year residents are still closely supervised, as attested to by surgeon William Nolen and pediatrician Claire McCarthy:

> An intern isn't expected to be a whiz kid. . . . There are plenty of others to provide the brainpower. What is needed from an intern is muscle and stamina. (22)

> Medical school teaches us a great deal, but supervised experience is necessary before we can go out on our own.
> I learned pediatrics [during my residency] the way I learned medicine during the last two years of medical school—as an apprentice, working under doctors senior to me. (xiv)

Nevertheless, first-year residents, still popularly called interns, now legally carry the title Doctor, and the significance of that designation weighs heavily on the conscience of most of them. Their sense of liminality may be at its greatest in those first two or three months of internship.

With internship comes a much larger patient load. From his or her first day, the intern is expected, among other things, to work much faster than just a month ago, to be the first physician to see patients admitted to a floor or to respond to an emergency when on call, and to teach medical students.

Exhaustion soon becomes a constant companion. Robert Marion's account of the morning *after* his first night on call captures the haze that wraps many a post-call resident:

> By concentrating all my efforts, I managed to finish the morning scut work by eight o'clock. While going about my chores, my exhausted mind continued to focus on one single fact: I needed to get out of there. I needed to get out of that neonatal intensive care unit or I would die. I had already begun to develop troubling symptoms: my breathing had become labored; I was inhaling and exhaling at least twice as rapidly as normal; my head was spinning and my belly aching. . . . So as soon as Terry Costa, the intern assigned to the next twenty-four-hour shift appeared at the front door of the NICU at a little after eight o'clock that morning, I approached her with an enormous sense of relief.
>
> "Congratulations," Terry said, smiling slightly as she walked briskly into the nurses' station. "You survived. You officially made it to your first weekend."
>
> "Oh, yeah, it's Saturday," I answered with all the strength I could muster. "Terrific." And with that, I burst into tears. (94)

For most interns, the call schedule not only defines the rhythms of a resident's life but also marks the measure of one's emotional limits. In recent years both the medical profession and some state laws have limited the number of consecutive hours that a resident (and some medical students) can work in the hospital. I shall consider the purpose and effects of these requirements in chapter 4.

Social and family life also fall under the power of call. Relationships are often portrayed as failing or surviving by virtue of a partner's ability to accommodate the intern's weariness, short temper, self-centeredness, and detachment. Craig A. Miller found that

> the only thing that had kept me sane during the long hours and constant humiliation had been the steady, calming support of my girlfriend. We'd been together for five years by this point, and it was a comfortable relationship, so the time seemed right to formalize things. I surprised her on Christmas morning with a marriage proposal, and she accepted. I did have some concerns, because I knew that the loneliness of a surgery resident's spouse is a matter of legend, and I wasn't sure how she would respond over the long haul. (27)

On Day 47 of her residency (in the late 1970s, one of the first part-time residencies in the country), a single mother, Michelle Harrison, records the pressures of solely carrying the responsibility for a child and their household:

> I thought I was okay yesterday, but I wasn't. I went home and thought of all the things I had to do, but I just collapsed. I was distressed that there weren't any groceries in the house, and I felt burdened by the whole household. I knew I was unreasonable, and went to bed. I got up for supper and went back to bed, and then got up about an hour later when Maggie's barking woke me. By then I was feeling better, but I was bothered because I knew I was reacting to the day, and that I had just kept everything inside. (111–12)

For interns who are childless or not part of a couple, there is equal despair over one's harried lot. Emily Transue finds herself one evening in a crowded bar:

> I would be hard-pressed to explain what I'm doing here, what brings me to a smoky, loud, meat-market nightclub at one o'clock on a Thursday morning, five hours before I have to be at work. I suppose I'm here because I'm twenty-five years old and the most rebellious thing I will have done with my twenty-sixth year, besides sharing a half dozen cigarettes, will be to call in sick for exactly one half day of clinic to go skiing. Because I'll feel guilty about that half-day. Because most nights that I'm not in the hospital I'm in bed asleep by ten, and most evenings that I have energy to do anything I spend at the gym, trying to prevent this life I have chosen from stealing my physical strength as it has stolen so much else. (74–75)

The personal and physical tolls of the internship resound in all accounts of this year, however rewarding the work may be.

Stories of patients account for the bulk of the writing, and some of the closest and most complicated relationships are described in this year. The exhaustion that interns take home with them also colors their lives and work with patients. Death continues to hover, always too near. I do not know of any physician who has written an unquestionably upbeat memoir about her or his internship. At the end of his memoir about this year, Stephen A. Hoffmann feels he has learned some important lessons about himself:

> Learning my limitations as a physician struck deeply at my self-esteem. . . .

When I emerged from internship, I felt badly wounded. Only now, [about six] years later, do I realize how much stronger I am for having discovered my limitations so soon. As doctors . . . [w]e must acknowledge and live with our mortal thoughts just as the people we treat learn to make do with diseases. We, too, are patients of sorts, and we are just as deserving of care. (299–300)

Many writers, like Robert Klitzman, find the entire year, upon its conclusion, to have a surreal air:

I had arrived in the hospital thirty-six hours earlier. After a night on call, no one bid me "thank you" for my toil. Now, no one said goodbye.

My mind was drained, and I felt weak. My legs barely held up my body. I walked into the white sunlight outside and gazed at people strolling up and down the sidewalk, looking healthy and free from IV poles. Familiar yellow taxicabs hurtled down the street uncaring. I had forgotten that the world still existed outside. I was surprised to see it, fresh, again. (222)

The internship is the most problematic year of a physician's education, both structurally and psychologically. Although most of the writers agree that it is important to learn to work under pressure, they also agree that too much pressure is unproductive, unnecessary, and even hazardous to interns and patients alike. Where that line is to be drawn, however, remains unclear.

POSTGRADUATE YEARS TWO THROUGH FIVE As residents pass through the succeeding years of postgraduate medical education, their level of responsibility grows, as does their comfort with that responsibility and the authority that accompanies it. The beginning of each new level of responsibility, however, often continues to give physicians pause. For example, as Danielle Ofri begins the second year of her residency she observes, "I hadn't been given any crash course on how to be a resident in charge. But it was the usual July 1st syndrome in which everyone was punted forward a notch. Like newborn piglets we wobbled forward into our new roles because there was no way to turn back the momentum. An intern was now standing before me in tears, entirely relying on me to save the day" (114). Toni Martin struggles to decide when and how, as a teacher, to delegate tasks responsibly: "It was physically impossible to perform every task as a resident, however, and those residents who tried cheated their charges of the learning experience. I agonized over how much to let the interns have their own heads, whether to allow tardiness on rounds, what were reasonable expectations of the students" (156–57). Even as the chief resident in neurosurgery, one of the longest residencies, Frank Vertosick Jr. reports the same initial queasiness, even liminality:

> As I drummed my fingers nervously on the table, I felt very alone. . . .
>
> The chief resident straddles two worlds. To the younger residents, the chief is just one more taskmaster who decides when they will take call, how many spinal taps they will perform, and what operative cases they are "ready" to do. To the attending staff, the chief stays a scut dog, a lackey who dances to their every whim. (253–54)

A minority of writers recount the full span of their residency. Those who do usually write much more selectively about landmark patients or events in the later years of residency. Writers often portray their responses to patients during these years as less volatile or judgmental than in earlier years. They often focus more on their professional styles or philosophies. Surgeon Elizabeth Morgan adopts what she considers a less "rigid" leadership style in the operating room. As she describes it, "I tried not to run a rigid service. I let Sean and the intern go home early when they could, and I tried to see we all got breakfast and dinner, when it was possible" (277). Emergency medicine physician Frank Huyler uses a spare prose style to set forth the complex interplay of what his patients see when they look at him, what they expect from him, how his work has shaped him, and his own sense of the immensity of that change in an essay titled "Time":

> Sometimes when I catch a glimpse of myself in a mirror, or reflected in a glass door, I understand why they're surprised when I enter the room. Their eyes widen. They often ask me.
>
> "I'm older than I look," I say, which is true. They're usually about ten years off when they guess. . . .
>
> I mind and I don't mind. When they see a kid in front of them, they don't want or expect it. They want the reassurance of age, the visible sign of experience. What they see disturbs them. They ask themselves, Is it possible? . . .
>
> Sometimes I'm angry. The kid with the bullet hole through the toe, slick black hair, shades, a thin angular face. Nine-millimeter, a party.
>
> "You're too young to be a doctor."
>
> He's seven years younger than I am. . . .

I like them when they are brave in the face of it. I like the old women who say they're ready, that they understand the surgery is dangerous, if they die they die. . . . I like the men who flirt with the nurses even though the EKG is unmistakable. . . .

It's late, and I go outside, stand in the entrance by the pneumatic doors, look to where the east lightens. I feel strong, but I know it won't last. . . . Something moves beside me, startling, and I turn. It's just the nurse, Susan, fumbling with her cigarettes.

"Not a bad night," she says, then adds the obligatory superstition. "So far." I nod and smile, watch the flare of the lighter and then the little coal at the tip of her cigarette, blooming as she takes a deep drag and lets the smoke out into the air. It twirls around us both, and we're quiet.

I'm thirty-two years old. (157–60)

"What they see disturbs them. They ask themselves, Is it possible?" Huyler writes here from his patients' perspective, but it is also his own. At the end the narrator marvels, albeit in an understated way, at what he has seen in the world, so much hardship and suffering, mindlessness and courage, in just a few years.

As with memoirs of undergraduate medical education and internship, those of the residency years conclude by taking stock. No writers come around to praising the educational process they have just completed, but they tend to be less heated in their criticism than those who focus only on the year of internship. Instead, many writers consider what they have learned about themselves and the medical profession. Some lessons are political. Steve Horowitz quotes from the lecture he delivered to incoming interns at the end of his residency—not the optimistic, encouraging speech his seniors had expected from him:

> You people have a responsibility that perhaps you're not even aware of. As you start your internships, you're going to become aware of inequities in the system. These inequities will include differences in care given to rich and poor people, and to black and white people. . . .
>
> Why am I so sure that ninety-nine out of one hundred will let things pass rather than rock the boat? The reason is that you people are a product of the system. You've been hand selected because you know how to play the game. . . . You may have beards and wear sneakers and try to impress people with how unconventional you look, but . . . you've gotten here by playing the game. (240–41)

Other lessons are personal. Emily Transue describes how she has learned to balance closeness and distance:

Stepping from a family meeting into the room of a sick ICU patient is like diving from air into water: the physical distance is so small, yet everything about the two worlds is intensely different. The thick emotional soup of the family meeting . . . There isn't room for [that] here.

Standing in the room I do not see his mangled face, his swollen, bloody lips. . . . He is a puzzle to be solved. He is physics and physiology.

Both of these worlds are familiar to me, comfortable in their way. I can hold a family member's hands and listen for the breathing change that shows they are about to cry. I can touch a shoulder and feel a grieving body shift its weight out toward my hand. And I can manage vents and float Swan-Ganz catheters and interpret arterial blood gases. In some perhaps twisted way, I enjoy both these things, but the magnitude of the transition will never cease to surprise and shock me. (225)

And some lessons are about medical education itself. Claire McCarthy begins her memoir with this assertion, and returns to it frequently as she describes her years from medical student to chief resident:

There are two components of medicine and its practice: the scientific and the emotional. The scientific is obvious and easily described; . . . the emotional is less obvious and more difficult to describe. . . .

There is a curriculum to teach the scientific component of medicine. . . . There is, however, no standard curriculum to teach the emotional component. . . .

I didn't expect the study of medicine to be quite as overwhelming and disturbing as it sometimes was. I didn't expect that part of becoming a doctor would be learning a culture of jargon, habits, and beliefs. I didn't realize that I would be learning not only how to do something, but how to be someone, someone I didn't always want to be. . . .

In so many situations what was required to help had nothing to do with drugs, surgery, or technology. The emotional component of medicine was incredibly pervasive and important, and it demanded more of me than I could ever have imagined. (xvi–xvii, xviii, xix)

As students and physicians move through the years of their medical education, the fire hose of information, stimulation, and expectations does not diminish. Most physicians find a way to drink what they need without completely drenching themselves, but most of the writers maintain a healthy skepticism about themselves and the claims of their profession. It is also important to remember that these writers continue to love the practice of medicine even when they chafe at its pedagogy. In the chapters that follow, I shall look more closely at these tensions between the goals and methods of medical education.

Embodiment

IN *A Not Entirely Benign Procedure* Perri Klass comments on two essays that she wrote at the end of her first two years of medical school: "I couldn't write either of those pieces now, even a couple of years later, because I have totally lost track of what it felt like" (29). In *The Cutting Edge*, Joni Lynn Scalia describes the chief of medicine as he appeared to the intimidated third-year students: "He was white and sterile and cold. He was sharp like a blade. He was the Future. The Mold. The Ultimate Cookie from which we were all to be cut" (4). Charles LeBaron, quoted in the introduction regarding his motivation to write *Gentle Vengeance*, worries about "a little vial of sweetness and kindness around stomach level" that he'd possessed before beginning medical school but now fears he might "spill . . . in wrath or discouragement" (268). And a photograph on the back of the dust jacket of John MacNab's *The Education of a Doctor* shows a young man in a slicker and rain boots mimicking the marching gait of a goose a few steps ahead of him—whether imprinting or learning to goose-step (neither particularly complimentary to medical education) is left to the viewer's interpretation.[1] Medical education is often talked about as a process of initiation, socialization, or professionalization, but the quotations and the image above suggest a transformation that is even more profound, a process that goes to the very core of the initiate's body.

None of the authors of these memoirs use the term *embodiment* in their writing, but a spate of scholarship in recent decades suggested it to me as I read these stories. To put it broadly, theories of embodiment are grounded in the observation that our understanding of ourselves and our world is filtered through our physical body. Similarly, how other people respond to our bodies affects how we, in turn, regard, treat, and present those bodies. The notion of embodiment challenges the long-oversimplified dualism of René Descartes' (in)famous proclamation, "I think, therefore I am." Although

Descartes never intended that his assertion about the power of conscious rationality create a permanent divide between mind and body, they have nevertheless become almost mutually exclusive in popular discourse, even though most people would readily acknowledge that this relationship is not quite so simple. Thus, in seeking to reestablish the codependence of mind and body, recent scholars in the humanities, sciences, and social sciences have brought new attention to the role that the body plays in social and personal identity. As literary historian and theorist Peter Brooks states, "Whatever it once was, the body is now problematic" (5).

Neurologists such as Antonio Damasio have studied how experience and memory register on and can alter the body at the cellular level, work that has been picked up by humanities scholars particularly interested in the effects of trauma on the human psyche.[2] Linguist George Lakoff and philosopher Mark Johnson relate language, human values, and the body by demonstrating the metaphorical nature with which the body imbues our most common words. For example, humans' *upright* position and usually *forward* gait evoke positive associations with these words wherever they appear: good behavior is generally "upright" and good progress is usually "forward" or "toward" a goal. Roland Barthes and Peter Brooks, drawing in turn on the postmodern theorists Jacques Lacan and Jacques Derrida, consider the relationship between an author's corporeality and the stories he or she writes. On the one hand, they have described the generation of language and stories as an inescapable distancing of the self from its body, as the process of *any* writing fosters intellectual contemplation of physical events. On the other hand, however, they also describe literature as the very expression of the body's desires, especially concerning vulnerability and mortality.[3] In this view, stories themselves attest to the embodied nature of creativity.

Other scholars challenge theories about gender, race, and sexuality that cast these phenomena as largely either biological or social. They criticize the former for locating identity too narrowly in a body over which its inhabitants have little or no control and the latter for leaving people stranded, so to speak, in a regulating world equally beyond their influence. Although both perspectives offer valuable insights into the forces that shape us, they often lead to generalizations that do not exactly match individuals' own backgrounds and personalities. In *Bodies That Matter* philosopher Judith Butler grapples with the complex interactions of biology, society, and individuality in her concept of *performativity*. She examines the historical concept of heterosexuality and the powerful cultural norms that have informed it. Butler's description of the performativity of gender can be applied to the cultural norms for "doctor" with useful results. Performativity is the aggregate of all those things a culture considers, in the instance of gender, to be masculine or feminine. There comes to be such widely held agreement about these appearances and gestures that they become social norms. Performativity is particularly visual, with the human body the medium by which gender is communicated. A person who identifies as "man" or "woman" usually adopts these norms and practices them until, after much repetition, he or she "becomes" masculine or feminine in the eyes of both self and others. The person becomes indistinguishable from the norms that define him or her as a man or a woman, "the effect of a dynamic of power, such that the matter of bodies will be indissociable from the regulatory norms that govern their materialization" (2).

If we substitute "doctor" for "man" or "woman," we would say that physicians in training practice the norms that define "doctor," norms held by physicians and patients alike (although they may not always be the same). To become comfortable as "doctor" it is necessary for effort*ful* performance to become effort*less* performativity, with an embodiment of the behaviors and attitudes that will be recognized by both patients and peers as "doctor." Performance is separate, different from performativity. Becoming a physician, then, is not only an intellectual but also a corporeal process, influenced by the norms that set boundaries for what "doctor" is.

Butler, however, does not see the process of achieving performativity as totally outside one's consciousness or will. Because heterosexuality is a historical norm, it is subject to "rearticulations" and resistance, by either groups of people or individuals who refuse to accept those norms and consciously perform against them (hopefully achieving a performativity of this new notion of gender or sexuality) (2). Similarly, "doctor" can be challenged, either individually or collectively. Norms can be repudiated, maybe even changed. But the social power behind those norms is formidable. It is this sense of a powerful, metaphorical sea change within themselves that the authors I cited at the start of this chapter sense. While they desire to become physicians, they are just beginning to realize what it means to be "doctor." Many of them will remain unaware that their bodies are sites on which this transformation is, uncomfortably, taking place.

This sweeping summary does scant justice to the meticulous, insightful work of many scholars. I shall expand more on some of these theories as my analysis progresses, but I am more interested here in a broader gestalt of embodiment and its consequences in physicians' work than in the subtleties of these sophisticated theories. In the discussion that follows, I shall catalog how the corporeal nature of medical education and practice becomes lodged in the physician's language and metaphors of memory, how the physical experiences of medical education register themselves on the student's body, how writers document their relationship to their own bodies and the bodies of patients, and how the physical work of medical education reveals the vulnerability that is an inherent part of becoming a physician.

Memory, Metaphor, and Performance

In *Lovestrong*, first-year medical student Dorothy Greenbaum dreams that a woman hails her as she is driving through the night:

> She stares at me through vacant eyes. Her skin is crisscrossed with red slashes. Her organs spill grotesquely in a pile on the pavement. It is the cadaver.
>
> "I felt *everything!*" she screams.
>
> I bolt up in bed, sweating and shaking. The early morning sun filters in through the blinds. I know that anatomy is over, but it will be a long time until I can distance myself from what I have seen. Once more I repeat Simon's words: "There are no ghosts in the anatomy lab." He was right. The ghosts were not in the lab. They were here, inside my head, waiting until I was ready to see them. (131)

Dreams are a frequent repository of memory in these memoirs, and nearly every author describes at least one of them (often a recurring one) that haunts, taunts, or chastises the dreamer.[4]

Peppered throughout the memoirs, however, are numerous comments, often no more than quick asides, that tie memory to sensation. In *Woman/ Doctor* Jane Patterson meets a man in a hospital hallway long after he had been her patient:

> His face lit up with pleasure. He was delighted that I had remembered him. After all, it had been more than ten years. In truth I would not have recognized him . . . had I not touched his hand. Once I touched him, I knew instantly. . . .
>
> Mr. Swartz had a degenerative collagen disease, scleroderma, that dries the skin and alters its texture. Touching the parchmentlike skin of his hand, I was transported instantly across the years." (208–09)

The words and images with which I opened this chapter represent medical education as a process that is inherently embodied; these passages lodge specific events of patient care in the physician's very brain, hands, and feet.

In *White Coat, Clenched Fist* Fitzhugh Mullan writes about his internship thus: "My recollections of Jacobi [Hospital] are dominated by the sensation of my baggy white uniform. . . . The laundry proved short on soap but well stocked with starch" (71). In *White Coat* Ellen Lerner Rothman writes, "My feet still remember the dull ache of long hours of standing in the operating room" (123–24). And, in *Under the Ether Dome*, Stephen A. Hoffmann describes how auditory memory serves to recall a pleasant time late one night when he was quietly sitting at the nurses' station writing in his patients' charts:

> A popular station was playing, and the music sounded unusually poignant and bittersweet, maybe because of the late hour or maybe because my state of awareness was heightened. As I read the charts and listened to the music, I felt a deep affection for my new world. In this affection were combined euphoria and an almost visceral longing, the kind that rises in the throat and borders on loneliness, and the feeling was made all the more profound by a pleasant sense of fatigue. . . . Throughout the first few months of my internship, music had this strange effect upon me late at night. Even now, when I reencounter the songs that were popular at that time, I relive, however briefly, this magic feeling. (38)

These writers also turn to their bodies when they seek metaphors to describe the effects of medical education. For example, in *Intern*, the pseudonymous Doctor X writes, "But for all his harassment and hurry, the intern *learns*. He absorbs knowledge through his skin. He learns lesson after painful lesson about the quirks and cruelties and surprises of human illness. Even more, he learns hard lessons in humility, patience, compassion and personal integrity" (13). The metaphor of learning as absorption through one's skin is an obviously embodied image of education, but the subsequent use of words such as "painful" and "hard" offers metaphor that is grounded in a physically vulnerable body, the kind of metaphor described by Lakoff and Johnson in which the physical and moral senses of a metaphor become almost inseparable. Sayantani DasGupta uses military in addition to other physical metaphors throughout *Her Own Medicine* to underscore her sense of the traditionally male violence that underlies medical education and practice: "The problem [of the harshness of medical education, particularly for women] is more imperceptible. It involves the subtle and not so subtle culture of medicine that seeps into a woman's skin only after she is well entrenched in the field" (4). Every memoir contains corporeal metaphors such as the following by, respectively, Dorothy Greenbaum and Charles LeBaron:

> Each one of those first patients has stayed with me. Each one was like the mark of a hammer on thin metal. I was neither better nor worse after the experience, just different—indelibly changed. (150)

> Mornings, when the weather's cold but clear, I run along the frozen paths of the Fenway. . . . I wonder if it will ever be my body again, with moments of flashing, mysterious poetry, not just a sack of enzymes, a matrix of lipoproteins, a jumble of hollow, pulsing viscera, a juicy computer where hard-wired, low-speed elements process frequency-coded voltage fluxes along phospholipid bilayers. (188)

The process implied by these metaphors goes beyond socialization: they imply a refashioning of the student's physical being.

I must remind readers here of two earlier qualifications I have made about these memoirs. First, undergraduate and graduate medical education for most students and residents corresponds with the years of their entrance into adulthood, which is an embodied, anxiety-provoking experience of its own; readers of these memoirs must be careful not to blame medical education for all of the writers' angst. Second, whatever criticisms most of these writers level at their education, most of them continue to hold the profession of medicine to high standards (hence their dismay or anger) and most of them choose to stay in medicine after completion of their residencies. Rhetorician Charles M. Anderson notes that students enter medical school desiring to wear the mantle of the physician. The stories they tell about their education often reflect *both* their "willing assimilation" into medicine and their "resistance" to the process (283). In other words, medical students want to be comfortable in a physician's environment *and* in a physician's body. Some students will accomplish this with little conflict, and the performativity of "doctor" will become a seemingly natural part of their demeanor. For some people, this seamless incorporation of "doctor" will never, or never completely, occur.

Medical students constantly wonder what kind of doctor they will "be," with "be" usually including their physical posture or demeanor. Some women students or residents are deliberately articulate on this point because of their awareness that they are working *against* the usual norms of "doctor." As she nears the end of her surgery residency, Elizabeth Morgan was quoted in the preceding chapter regarding her efforts to avoid running a "rigid service." She goes on to say, "I was evolving my own style of being a surgeon—considerate of my team whenever that was possible" (277). For both men and women, "doctor" feels more like a performance in the early years of their education. Even before they learn how to execute a single medical procedure, students experience the tension between how patients expect doctors to act and how they feel capable of acting. Wearing a white coat and often introduced to patients as Doctor So-and-So makes students uncomfortable about a deception that to them exceeds their right. For example, as she prepares to outfit herself to see patients, Dorothy Greenbaum chooses a metaphor of physical growth to describe her worries:

> I began to experience a disturbing confusion. I wasn't really a doctor, yet I would be working with patients, treating illnesses, spending all my time with the hospital staff. In preparation for this clerkship, my professors had stressed the importance of professional confidence. They had made a point of saying that for some of us, "Doctor" would be a title we would have to grow into. They were right. My "growing pains" began as I stood staring at the blank name tags. (134)

The physician's white coat often becomes a site for the tension that accompanies conscious performance. Ellen Lerner Rothman notes, with symbolic irony, that she was given a coat "several sizes too large" at the start of her medical education (2). The white coat has power not only over the patients who encounter it but also over the wearer, as Emily Tranuse observes about her resident's coat (traditionally longer than the short jacket of medical school): "The long coat is synonymous with authority, with competence. The coat seems stronger than my own persona, I try to become the person who is wearing it. I notice myself adjusting my posture, my bearing, to match the coat. I occasionally allowed myself a certain frivolity as a student, which seems inappropriate in this new attire. Act your age, the coat seems to insist. You are a doctor now" (6). Judith Butler writes about the norms that dictate sexual identity and the power they can wield over individuals. Medical students are often painfully aware of the norms that define "doctor" and the power of the expectations that are beginning to be imposed on them—and that they are beginning to impose upon themselves.

Stephen A. Hoffmann makes fun of his insecurity about his appearance as he deliberately stages a performance that feels unnatural to him:

Having studied the attire of a junior resident who had been on duty [in the emergency ward] the day before, I copied his example, tying a rubber tourniquet around one belt loop and affixing a pair of EKG calipers to another. A reflex hammer, I had learned from watching a neurologist, could be kept conveniently in a buttonhole of my white coat, and a safety pin, which I would use to test sensation, fit neatly through one of the coat's lapels. I studded my pockets with scissors and tape and tucked in several intravenous catheters where I could still find room. Preparing for each rotation of the year, as every intern knows, is very much a matter of looking *and becoming one* with the part. (158–59, my italics)

In striking contrast, Joseph Sacco describes the distraught body of a first-year resident (that is, an intern) who learned how to play the part of the humane, skilled physician implied by the white coat, even when the mind of its inhabitant is barely there:

I suppose that in the end I *behaved* like someone who cared, I went through the *motions* of someone who did good, I did what I understood to be the *right thing* for all my patients because I knew that not doing so would turn me from a "caring doc" into a "bad doc." Maybe I *did good* because I feared failing the teachings of my upbringing, and becoming the kind of doc that society, in its two-faced way, frowned upon. Maybe the dead bright-eyed guy would one day wake up, and I'd be glad I'd done good because once again it would be important to me for its own sake.

Nonetheless, let me assure you that as an intern, I really didn't care. (183)

Sacco describes himself as being aware of two people, a "caring doc" and a "bad one," whose behaviors are judged by a "dead bright-eyed guy" whose conscience is guided by the values of his youth and his awareness of what society expects him to be, even when another level of his being does not share those feelings. Here, body becomes dissociated from emotion (or the lack of emotion), a physical buffer between the vulnerable patient and the hazardous intern.

Beneath the white coat, medical students sometimes mark their bodies with their ambivalence about the kind of physician they believe their teachers expect them to become. In *Heart Failure* Michael Greger protests against a humorless, regimenting notion of medical practice. Early in his pediatrics clerkship, Greger delights a child by painting her fingernails:

and she paints mine—a lovely purple-brown. I wore them to rounds this morning.

My senior resident took me aside. "Your fingernails are getting in people's way," he said. Huh? "The attendings are complaining; this is a conservative profession." Defensively, I tried to explain that I didn't paint them myself, mad that I even felt the need to explain at all. He knew. He knew that she had done it. He replied, "Medicine is also an anti-emotion profession."

She gets to do my toenails tonight. (14–15)

And she does. In the last entry of his diary, Greger writes, "I sit down on our bed and rub my feet, toenail clipper in hand. It is said that tectonic plates— whole continents—move as fast as nails grow. I pause, and squeeze off the last chipped crescent of that lovely purple-brown" (97). The "lovely" polish on his toes sustains Greger both immediately and metaphorically through a seemingly endless third year. With the clipping of the last bit of paint, Greger suggests an invisible, permanent change deep within himself, of which he does not have total control, as if some part of himself has now become performative, lodged out of reach but within his own physical being.

Other writers depict the emphasis on appearance with irony and poignance. Jane Patterson, one of the few woman interns in the late 1960s, chose her look with care:

I was, I think, a particularly laughable figure in those days. I had assiduously cultivated a no-nonsense, authoritative air, reinforced by a hairdo in which every lock was pulled back from my face, straight and severe, and coiled into a precise bun dead center atop my head. . . . It was a look I thought befitting a woman doctor. I affected a brisk, efficient manner and spoke in clipped tones. I was a terribly important, terribly busy, terribly competent person. . . . But there were those glasses. I had, after much internal debate, traded my sensible, horn-rimmed glasses in for a pair of those plastic-framed affairs popular at the time (at least among certain sets), the kind that had wing tips, rather like the tailfins on old Cadillacs, swooping up from the outer edges of the frame on either side. Highlighting this lovely look was a spray of rhinestones embedded in the plastic of the wing tips. I thought them madly elegant and imagined that they added a touch of feminine glamour to my image. (I had, in those days, a great deal of imagination.) (119)

Fitzhugh Mullan writes about a third-year classmate, Jim Waller, the only student in 1966 sporting a beard into his clerkships:

> [Waller] received a terse note from the Dean of Students requesting him to shave. The news of the demand spread quickly through the class, angering many people. . . . The idea that some medical school bureaucrat could dictate my hair style and dress as well as what I studied and how many hours of my life I spent in the hospital and how I spent my summers . . . was the last straw, the unacceptable excess in the invasion of my privacy as a human being."[5]

And, in her qualitative study of African American women surgeons, Patricia L. Dawson records instances in which female medical students are aware of their tenuous position as either a woman or an African American. Xena (her assigned name for the interview) describes her emotional experience as being affected by her physical appearance, emphasizing how the body is inseparable from the phenomenon of racial and gender discrimination:

> I would say residency was hard. I think it was more difficult because of the color of my skin and that relates to not having someone that I could identify with. They don't have to be your friend, but someone you can identify with so that you can make some connection and say, OK, well, this is how this works.
>
> You're always second-guessing yourself, because you never see your face on the other side. I think the ability to see yourself there as a woman—as an African American woman—not feel like you're going to be dodging bullets, would make it a lot better.
>
> I think that in the world, as human beings, we ask ourselves, "What is our purpose?" and you look to see yourself someplace. (84)

From the earliest days of medical school, students are aware of the performative concessions required to become a physician, but they try to negotiate some of the terms in ways better suited to their personal styles and values. Throughout these memoirs, the authors grapple to articulate and enact identities as physicians both within and against the expectations and examples set before them. In short, they strive to create a *performance* that holds the least amount of dissonance between how they see themselves as individuals-who-would-be-physicians and how their patients, teachers, and an amorphous "public" defines "doctor." In this way, they try to keep open the door through which, Butler suggests, change or individual resistance occurs. The authors cited at the start of this chapter fear losing this awareness.

Vulnerability

These metaphysical debates between one's self and one's self-as-physician reveal the complex dynamic of body, culture, and psyche in the shaping of a professional identity. But it is in the day-to-day descriptions of medical education that the writers reveal the extent of their own body's engagement in becoming "doctor." Memoirs of medical education abound with sensory description and at times even seem to revel in the lurid or scatological. Medicine has always been a profession that depends on the senses, a dependence that has always been in league and in tension with the rise of medical technologies.[6]

Visual images are the most common: the unnatural pallor of cadavers in gross anatomy and autopsy labs, the virulent red and white of blood and protruding bone in the emergency room, the stark lights and draped forms of the operating room, the ghostly halls or tunnels of a hospital at night. However, the other senses are drawn upon as well. Audrey Young notes smell: "For a moment I smelled the acidic stink in the room again and my stomach turned. Later I would identify the smell as amniotic fluid and smell the fluid on my scrubs and in my hair, and in the steam of a shower after a long night in the hospital" (55). Frank Huyler records sound: "He was in his early forties, and all he did as he lay on the hospital bed was chew pieces of ice. After a while I came to identify that sound—the crunch of teeth on ice—with him" (15). And William Nolen remarks upon taste: "One of the M.E.'s [medical examiners, performing an autopsy] even smoked a cigar when he worked, resting it occasionally on the slab and then nonchalantly popping it back into his mouth. I could hardly bear to watch him" (110). Each of these brief descriptions not only evokes a smell, sound, or taste but also registers it within the writer's body, underscoring sensation as a phenomenon *received into* the body as well as *perceived by* it. (Physicians' memoirs are not alone in such visceral prose. Although much fewer in number, nurses' memoirs of education and early practice are probably even more graphic—and often written to trace the trajectory of burnout, suggesting that the norm of nurse as a bottomless well of selfless caring can deny the emotional effects of such work on the nurse him- or herself.)[7]

After sight, the sense most often evoked is touch. Although some critics complain that medicine is dangerously replacing touch with technology, students still learn the basics of sensation and palpation in the physical examination of patients. Learning, for example, how to "take a pulse" or "appreciate the liver" are sources of anticipation and pride for students, but physical contact in diagnosis and treatment can also be a source of anxiety. Anxiety about touching a patient is often cast as a fear of hurting him or her, an anxiety that usually dissipates as students become more adept at performing procedures and talking to patients. Perri Klass was quoted in the preceding chapter about her comfort with apologizing for drawing a patient's blood, reasoning that "however necessary the pain may be, I am not the one who has to bear it." Authors remain aware of the thin line between therapy and assault. Joseph Sacco uses as many tactile verbs as possible to describe what he believes to be the torture endured by patients in the effort to keep them alive at any cost:

> As far as I'm concerned, the left- or right-wing moralist is welcome to come into the hospital and stab the patient seven to ten times a day for blood, shove a tube into his penis for a specimen of urine, into his nose for a gob of infected snot, into his stomach for feeding, and into his mouth to unclog a blocked airway. The moralist can, without the patient's or the family's specific written or verbal consent, irradiate the patient daily for chest X-rays, poke him twice or thrice a day to replace his IV and, when the patient codes, break his ribs doing chest compressions, shove a tube into his trachea, and bayonet his thighs for arterial blood. In fact, if he wants, he can cut the patient's chest open and manually squeeze the heart to maintain a pulse. (253)

Sacco's moral outrage with the extremes of resuscitation is depicted by language that reflects not only the violence being done *to* a patient's body but also the violence being done *by* a physician's body.

Touch can also create a positive psychological connection, at least for the practitioner. In *Learning How the Heart Beats* Claire McCarthy describes an experience from her years as an undergraduate medical student:

> She looked so pale, so frightened. I stood watching her for a few moments. Suddenly I realized what I could do.
>
> I reached over and put my hand on hers. "You can squeeze my hand if you want," I said.
>
> She looked at me. She didn't say anything, but she nodded ever so slightly and let go of the side of the table. I took her hand in mine; she squeezed it, hard. . . .

I asked the woman about her classes. I felt stupid as soon as I asked. . . .
But the woman's eyes relaxed a little, and she answered readily. In short
sentences interrupted by wincing, she listed her classes for me and said
she was having trouble with her statistics course. Each time she winced
she squeezed my hand a little harder. . . .

[At the end of the procedure, the] woman sat up as the intern brought
in the wheelchair. It wasn't until we were helping her off the table that I
realized I was still holding her hand. (77–78)

Stephen A. Hoffmann, quoted in the preceding chapter, memorializes one
of his patients by carrying a vial of the young man's blood in the pocket
of his white coat, finding some solace in the very tactile nature of the act:
"Suspended at his side, I was at a loss for what to do. His presence seemed to
demand some reaction, especially *since my hands enclosed a sample of his blood,*
a sample *that was still warm*. . . . Throwing it away was out of the question.
Instead, I placed the tube in one of the pockets of my white coat and *held
it there* for almost a week. It was the only substitute for a memorial I could
devise" (183, my italics).

Next to touching the body of a patient, the most frequent descriptions of
touch involve body fluids. Joseph Sacco writes,

> I began to sweat the sixth or seventh layer of sweat I had shed in the pre-
> ceding twenty or so hours. In the next fifteen or sixteen hours I would
> sweat a good eight or ten layers more. Each would capture and lock next
> to my body the particular odor, be it shit, piss, or vomit, characterizing
> the location in which I was sweating, along with the all-pervasive, sharp
> smell of ammonia-based disinfectant. (15)

For Jane Patterson, the "feel"—physically, cognitively, and emotionally—of
a patient's blood or one's own sweat soaks through to her deepest fears and
darkest despair about the limits of medicine and of herself as a physician:

> Maybe it wouldn't have been quite so bad, maybe we could have pretended
> that all the vomit and blood soaking through our clothes right down to our
> underwear at some ungodly hour of the morning was worth it because a
> life was being saved, except that in a week or a month the same old gomer
> would be back again, vomiting blood and screaming obscenities as a tube
> was being stuffed down his throat. It didn't feel a bit like Ben Casey or
> Florence Nightingale. (30)

Frank Vertosick Jr. links the numbing work of the lowly intern in surgery with the actual numbing of his fingers during cardiac surgery: "Our purpose was to take night calls and to be human retractors in the operating room. During the day, I held quivering hearts upside down so that a vein graft could be sewn into their backsides. Immersed in iced saline during cardiopulmonary arrest, the hearts froze my fingers, and only hours after surgery did my frostbitten fingers regain their feeling" (51–52).

Writers of such descriptions often connect such sensations with being physically soiled. Dorothy Greenbaum describes her disheveled, soaked, and swollen body as she limps, alone, to her car, before dawn:

> I am dressed in my surgical greens. My ankles swell over the tops of my sneakers, which are stained with purple dye, Betadine and blood. My hair is matted with heat and perspiration, and the scent of my body merges with the odor of alcohol, disinfectant and benzoin. The hospital smells have become a personal perfume I carry with me. Some nights they linger, following me as I make my way toward the darkened parking lot and home. (11)

Memoirs of medical education and residency are replete with descriptions of bodies that struggle to keep themselves clean, nourished, rested, relaxed, and physically fit. Eating is frequently squeezed into stolen moments: "Unable to relax, I eat my supper standing up. Pacing with my soup," Michael Greger writes (26). As an intern, Robert Klitzman slips into the ward's walk-in refrigerator at 5 A.M.:

> A cloud of cold, wet vapor enveloped me. . . . I felt frozen and numbed in the surgical scrub suit I wore when on call. The low V-neck of the loose shirt stuck to my chest. The baggy pants clung to me, weighed down by a heavy beeper. . . .
> *Room* 919, it read. *McDonald.*
> I pulled the tray out all the way, and weighed it in my hands. It would have been her last supper. I looked down at the plastic cutlery, the covered main dish. . . .
> I had been reduced to a scavenging beast, an automaton. My intellect still functioned, though at a slightly slowed speed. I was emotionless and guiltless, barren and icy. Survival first. . . .
> It was the coldest meal I ever ate. (100–01)

Steve Horowitz remembers bladders and bowels that must be disciplined: "Almost twenty hours had elapsed and I hadn't taken a piss. Up until now I hadn't needed to. I think it must be some type of yoga. . . . A good physician, I think, never has to take a crap during a cardiac arrest" (26–27).

Personal fitness often falls by the wayside. Theodore Isaac Rubin tracks the rise and fall of his weight during his four-month rotation in the emergency room: "This guy is thirty-five and is sure as shit an excellent candidate for a C.V.A. or coronary. But who am I to talk—I'm up to 250 again, and this, too, is surely self-destructive as hell and I don't need analysis to know that. I got to get my ass into the dieting sling as of this A.M. for sure and STAT!" (114). Blogger Brandon Barton vows, "The senior [medical student] and I are planning to lose weight and read a lot this month, we will encourage each other hopefully. Time for sleep!"[8]

The other side of the coin in maintaining a healthy body appears in frequent reports of institutions' disregard for their charges' health. In *Learning to Play God* Robert Marion responds scornfully to the physician who pronounces him to be "in excellent health":

> I wasn't in excellent health that day; I wasn't even in good health. I was fat, having gained over fifteen pounds during the time I'd been in Boston. I was out of shape, since I hadn't had time for exercise, other than my walks between the bus stop and the medical center, for the entire previous year. I was chronically overtired, overstressed, and overburdened, and my spirit and my heart had been broken. But none of this was uncovered in the physical exam the health service doctor performed. (185)

Joni Lynn Scalia writes angrily about the lack of consideration she was given when diagnosed with diabetes during her internship, and Lisa Iezzoni describes how she was discouraged from pursuing a residency because of her diagnosis with multiple sclerosis.[9] In recent years, however, Brandon Barton has written openly about taking Paxil for anxiety,[10] and Ron Maggiore has described being provided with a paper-and-pencil exam instead of a computer-based one because of his history of seizure disorder.[11] Little, though, is known about the numbers or experiences of medical students and residents with disabilities, a further indication that the physician's body and its performance are still powerfully regimented and expected to be as strong and invulnerable as his or her mind. The writers of these memoirs struggle to determine when this strength is truly necessary and when it can prove detrimental to both physician and patient.

The pregnant body and motherhood do not generally appear in the memoirs until the mid-1980s, but they quickly become, if not commonplace, at least not especially noteworthy. In *Baby Doctor* Perri Klass writes about listening to a "famous NICU [neonatal intensive care unit] resuscitation story" while pregnant. It is a grisly tale of deeds done in direct denial of the parents' wishes: "I got furious. I wrapped my arms around my belly, thinking of the fetus inside, still a secret from my colleagues. What was in my belly was *mine*. . . . And I rubbed my belly and promised the baby inside, you come out tonight, you die in my arms. No neonatologists will get anywhere near you" (300–01). Women *and* men who are parents often recognize themselves in their patients or the patients' families. Claire McCarthy's observation is representative of many of the male writers as well: "As the mother swayed she rubbed the baby's back, gently, rhythmically. I felt a rush of recognition. This was how I so often held Michaela" (241). Conversely, some women who have not experienced childbirth write about their discomfort in the labor and delivery room. Ellen Lerner Rothman writes, "The grossness bothered me because I knew I would be in labor too someday" (173). Students' and residents' experiences of gender, as well as race and other forms of difference, is an immense subject, which I shall say more about in the next chapter. It must suffice here to say that embodying oneself as a physician does not supersede a person's other embodied identities. Indeed, conflicting social or cultural views about these various identities may only make the performance of any one of them more confusing or stressful.

Physicians in training also discover that their bodies can feel threatened by patients. Sometimes, sexuality threatens. Melvin Konner describes the response an unsuspecting patient elicits in him:

As in most neurological examinations, there was no reason to intrude on any part of the body ordinarily considered intimate, and of course I did not. But I soon found out that any part of the body is intimate in the sense that it is protected by the customary barriers of interpersonal space. . . .

My task was greatly complicated by the fact that I was doing my very first physical examination on a woman who promptly aroused in me unmistakable if fleeting feelings of romantic tenderness and sexual desire. . . .

The simplest things—looking into her mouth, testing the suppleness of her neck, pushing down on her knee to test the muscle strength in her thighs, checking the mobility of her ankle joint—seemed almost intolerably intrusive. Touching the neck or the knee of a beautiful woman was something one earned with an appropriate investment of time and sentiment. (31)

In other situations, these writers describe the potential for physical harm from their patients, most often as vectors of infection. When Audrey Young realizes that HIV/AIDS is a possible diagnosis for one of her patients, she responds, "Now I could feel the warmth of Virgil's body just a few feet away and I felt something inside of me step back slowly from him" (31). Forty years earlier, William Nolen commented, "I didn't want to carry tubercule bacilli from one patient to another of course, and this was one reason I was extremely careful; the other reason, a more selfish one, was that I certainly didn't want to acquire active T.B. myself" (151). Writers occasionally report fearing physical force from patients or their families. Danielle Ofri describes one such instance with a patient's aunt: "I tried to edge backward, but she locked her glare on me and I couldn't move. Her angry breath seared the skin on my face. 'I don't trust you,' she said, plunging one firm finger into my chest. 'Stay away from my niece!'" (173). Compared to all depictions of contact with patients, however, concerns about an author's physical safety are very much in the minority.

By far the greatest physical hardship reported in these memoirs is lack of sleep. The assault begins in the first weeks of medical school, as documented by online diarist Brian Hartman:

> Really nothing much to add. I had a glass of wine with studying so I'm all relaxed and will try to crash. I took a two-hour nap around 6pm though so I'm not sure how easily sleep will come. I wonder if I have sleep apnea because I never seem to be rested, even after nine hours of sleep. Hrm.

Lack of sleep follows most students into their clinical rotations, as it did Toni Martin: "Lots of times [at home] you barely get through dinner before you crash" (99). The most extreme descriptions of exhaustion, however, come from the early years of residency. Robert Marion's description of his physical symptoms post-call were quoted in the preceding chapter, and other writers go on to attest to a spectrum of hazards that can result from lack of sleep. William Nolen notes "emotional instability" wrought by "those long hours," remembering one particular instance: "By Saturday morning at eight, I was on the verge of hysteria. I didn't even feel tired any more, just hyper. I thought I was functioning beautifully, though I'm certain, in retrospect, that I couldn't have been. I'm sure I was a mess" (80). Craig A. Miller writes about his decreased competence as a tired physician: "I was primarily forgetful of details. I was also embarrassingly inefficient. I can still vividly recall . . . leaf[ing] through the order book under the flickering fluorescent lights at the nurse's station, then star[ing] down in disbelief at the completed handwritten order, with my signature attached. I had already written the order hours before, but now had no recollection of having done so at all" (30).

Such dangerous levels of exhaustion can trigger a frightening sequence of events, traced in greater detail in chapter 4, that begins with a loss of compassion—

> It was only 7:00 P.M., but I had been awake for sixty hours and I wanted to go home and to sleep. Curtly I told him to at least try to answer my questions. He timidly answered each question after that, looking frightened. . . . When I went home I felt so guilty for being unkind that I couldn't sleep, and I planned in the morning to be especially nice to him.[12]

—descends into self-pity—

> The night after being on call was in some ways worse than the call night itself. The hospital that had swallowed me up for thirty-six hours then spat me out into the fading daylight. On the way home I glared at all the people on the street; everyone looked at me as merely another person on his way home from work. No one seemed to be aware of how special I was for having spent a horrible but heroic day-and-a-half at the hospital. The traffic didn't part, and I wasn't ushered through red lights—it didn't seem fair.[13]

—and deteriorates to blaming the patient:

> Then I asked [the resident], "So, what happened?"
> He replied, "He bleed and bleed and bleed and keep pulling out IV from thrashing around in bed."
> I said, "Why was he thrashing around in bed?" and he said, "Because he have big-time case of hepatic encephalopathy and go completely crazy."
> I asked, "So what wound up happening?"
> The resident replied, "I tie him down so he can't pull out IV anymore and he keep bleeding and throwing up blood and finally die at about eight in the morning without letting me sleep at all."[14]

The resident's mimicry of the patient's dialect heightens his illogical cruelty, but his account is representative of a scenario depicted with outrage and shame in many of these memoirs. Among the "laws" of *The House of God*, Samuel Shem's cult novel, admittedly highly autobiographical, are "AT A CARDIAC ARREST THE FIRST PROCEDURE IS TO TAKE YOUR OWN PULSE" and "THEY CAN ALWAYS HURT YOU MORE" (178, 88). The language of these two laws captures both the physician's own physiological response to a patient's medical danger and the jaded resident's belief that a patient can and can desire to inflict bodily harm on his or her doctors. Paradoxically, the student's or resident's or *any* physician's fear of personal vulnerability, whether physical or psychological, can lead to abuses of power of which the practitioner is at least temporarily oblivious.

Performing Vulnerability

All these episodes reveal the vulnerability of both patient *and* practitioner. These are stories about transgression, and they are usually written in conjunction with an author's story of his or her struggle to renegotiate the moral terms of "doctor." In *Hot Lights, Cold Steel* orthopedic surgeon Michael J. Collins tells one such story that is particularly rife with language and metaphors that underscore the embodied nature of his educational and developmental ordeal. Collins's story begins when Ben, a sixteen-year-old boy, is brought into the emergency room after his arm was torn off by a farming machine. He was probably dead upon arrival, but the surgical team "pumped him full of blood, shot him full of drugs, flailed away with CPR, clamped and cauterized various unrecognizable strands of vessels in the stump" (149). The senior resident eventually stops the resuscitation, and "as usual," Collins writes, "I had no time to think about what had just happened" (150). Eight hours later, though, when he returns to the call room at 4 A.M., he cannot relax:

> Everything inside me seemed to have been beaten away. I wasn't tired. I wasn't depressed. I wasn't sad, or outraged, or horrified. I was just empty. I kept seeing the gaping hole where Ben's shoulder should have been. I kept feeling guilty that Ben's death was another step on my learning curve, another item on my résumé. I needed things like that to become a surgeon. They brought me a step closer to my goal.
>
> The whole thing made me sick. I wondered if any goal could be worth all this. It wasn't that I minded the work. In some ways the mind-numbing drudgery was my salvation. It was a crutch, a shield. I got tied up in it and

it insulated me, protected me. It used me, but I used it, too; and I had drifted into a comfortable marriage with it. I immersed myself in work in order to distort and disguise what I did.

That was not a human being my scalpel was slicing through. It was a knee. No, not a knee but a meniscus. No, not a meniscus but a target, a single unit of focus upon which my attention could be riveted. (151)

Collins continues his use of metonymy as he relives the surgery he performed on Ben:

My bloody hand, removing the last shred of Ben's brachial plexus, was neither bloody nor mine. The plexus was neither severed nor brachial. It was merely a white target in a red-black hole. I could avoid the implications of my actions by ignoring the context in which they took place. They were isolated acts, devoid of meaning or greater significance. But I couldn't deceive myself forever. The hand that emerged from that gaping wound was not the hand that had entered it, and the eyes that finally turned away from that mangled corpse were not the eyes that first registered the gory scene. (152)

Collins's "bloody hand" represents his whole surgical being, but it marks his emotional dissociation from the act his body is performing. He describes a process of deliberate disembodiment in which both the patient's body and his hand become so objectified that they provide a shield to his consciousness: "We are not meant to see sixteen-year-old kids die" (152). Collins takes his shaving kit into the call room's bathroom, but finds he "had no interest in seeing the face in the mirror," his choice of an article over a pronoun further sealing his dissociation from himself (152).

Collins's soliloquy turns to his sense of isolation from teachers he has formerly admired and who profess a posture he can no longer sustain. He imagines being chastised by his residency director, B. J. Burke:

"An orthopedic resident is supposed to practice orthopedics, Doctor. He is not supposed to go around asking patients if they have ever considered the ontological implications of their fragile, mortal state."

"I didn't exactly—"

He jumps to his feet and points his finger at me. "We fix things. Do you understand that? . . . If somebody wants to be analyzed they can see a shrink. When they come to the Department of Orthopedics at the Mayo Clinic they want only one thing: they want to be fixed.

"Now get the hell out of here and go fix things. And I better not get any more reports of touchy-wouchy, hand-holding sessions in this department." (153)

Just when he should be achieving performativity as "doctor," Collins's own body conspires with his conscience to question medicine's precepts, as represented by B. J. Burke.

Over the next several years Collins struggles, alone, keeping his heretical notions to himself. Two years later, he is the senior resident when Kenny Johannson, a fourteen-year-old boy who has been run over by a tractor, is brought to the hospital: "I lifted the sheet covering the lower half of his body, and immediately the thick, fetid stink of manure mushroomed up at me. . . . The jagged end of the tibia stuck through a rent in his dirty blue jeans. A spreading pool of blood soaked the sheet underneath him" (286). Less than an hour later Kenny disappears—"On the surgical field in front of me was a leg" (289)—but this time Collins does not disassociate Kenny's body or his own surgical hand:

> Did we really think by hanging sterile blue sheets in a room on the second floor of a hospital we were no longer required to think of those things, too?
>
> This was not some abstract problem of surgical technique or diagnosis. This was not even a dispassionate analysis of the viability of muscle tissue or the regenerative ability of nerves. This was deciding whether to amputate a kid's leg. This required an understanding that an amputation means more than just severing bone, muscle, and tendon. This required an understanding of what a scalpel can and can't do. (289)

Collins considers that he could "fix the kid's leg" rather than amputate it. He possesses the skill to perform such an operation, but as the surgery progresses he sees that such surgical pyrotechnics would prove futile within a few months. He considers that, because this is the last night of his residency, he could perform the miracle that Kenny hopes for and leave someone else "to do the dirty work." Collins weighs the chance to do a complicated, exciting procedure and look like a hero against his sense of accountability to Kenny and Kenny's family as well as to himself. Only after all of these factors have contributed to his surgical decision does he allow himself to transform Kenny's leg into a mechanical object:

I looked at the mutilated pile of skin and bone that up until two hours ago had been a miracle of functioning flesh. Now it was only a mass of dark meat lying on a blue surgical sheet slowly oozing its life away.

I picked up a scalpel and began the amputation. (290)

Collins has written this account of his professional evolution with very specific moral landmarks that may not have occurred so exactly—or so obviously—at the time. Of all the memoirs in my study, this one seems to have had the longest time between the experiences and the writing (somewhere between twenty and twenty-five years, guessing from some cultural and historical references Collins makes). Collins, in fact, begins his memoir with a prologue, in italics, of the frenzied moments leading up to his decision to amputate Kenny Johannson's leg: "No one moved. No one spoke. They all waited" (xii). Nearly three hundred pages unfold before Collins takes his readers back to this moment, underscoring the importance that decision came to hold for him. In the course of crafting the comparison of his responses to Ben (significantly, Collins does not give Ben a last name) and Kenny Johannson, Collins traces his changing conscience and self-confidence. He has discovered that his vulnerability as a physician lies not in his technical competence but in the danger of thinking of his patient *and* of himself only as mechanisms without a future in a social world. He concludes that his own sense of moral vulnerability is a necessary condition for being the kind of doctor he can live with. Ironically, it was Collins's own vulnerability, experienced both mentally and physically, that allowed him to avoid becoming the kind of performative "doctor" his culture prescribed.

I do not know whether Collins articulated this insight so completely at any of the moments he describes in the course of this experience. At whatever point he achieved this understanding of his own moral base for making decisions, he is not equally explicit about the embodied nature of his development. On the whole, however, none of the writers of these memoirs recognize the extent to which their physical selves have participated in their growth into the identity of "doctor." Even though the memoirs of medical students and young physicians are remarkable for their sensory detail, the writers never comment upon the extent to which they absorb their professionalism through their very pores.

This should not be surprising. Given the frequency with which students and residents receive direct or indirect messages to be physically and emotionally tough, it is little wonder that the language and images of embodiment seldom receive direct attention in their memoirs. Emotions themselves, often dismissed as irrational (e.g., a *gut* feeling, *heart*-wrenching), also inhabit the world of the body, further assuring their dismissal by medical students and physicians. The repeated denial of the physical needs of a physician by teachers and even their peers may render this inexorable relationship invisible or inarticulable to the students and residents undergoing the vulcanization that produces the unflappable "doctor." Perhaps seeing oneself as physically vulnerable makes physicians feel more like their patients than they care to. Most of these writers deplore the distance between physician and patient that medical education seems to produce. They write, however, about an emotional or intellectual distance, rather than a physical one.

The physical vulnerability of both patient and physician seems to offer a valuable starting point for thinking about the privileges and responsibilities of being a physician. Recognizing the embodied nature of the practice of medicine opens a new dimension for understanding one's development as a physician and the work of medicine itself. Acknowledging one's physical vulnerability as a practitioner can, perhaps, foster narcissism or self-pity, but only if vulnerability is seen as weakness. Accepting the idea that medicine is, inevitably, an embodied profession and that *all* bodies are vulnerable can also foster humility, promote emotional honesty, and support a more healthful process of medical education.

Power and Difference

THE MOST COMMON criticisms of medicine and medical education have to do with power. Most discussions center around differences between physicians and their patients. Power is often granted to physicians by virtue of their specialized knowledge. Physicians are often more socially powerful than their patients in terms of their incomes and cultural backgrounds. There are, however, also power differentials *within* the medical profession, likewise based on differences in knowledge, status, and cultural background. Medical education is subject to these same biases, but people who write memoirs about their experiences also record three unanticipated phenomena related to power. First, upon entering medical school, they discover that friends and even family members now regard them with a new deference, a distinction they find both flattering and isolating. Second, students quickly discover that they are at the bottom of a medical pecking order through which they must painstakingly advance. Some writers go on to note that, however low they may reside in the order, patients "can also be found at its most subterranean level, below even the subbasement of the medical students."[1] Even so, many of these writers record a third phenomenon: a process by which they come to see themselves as powerless pawns at the mercy of their own teachers *and* patients.

The concept of power has long been studied by scholars across the humanities and social sciences. In thinking about the roles of difference and power in medical education, I have been particularly influenced by the French historiographer Michel Foucault, physician and philosopher Howard Brody, and physician and sociologist Howard Waitzkin, whose precepts I outline very briefly here. In *The History of Sexuality* Michel Foucault introduced the notion of *the other* in tracing the cultural history of homosexuality.[2] "Other" is the social position held by those men and women whose behavior (or even existence) has been deemed as outside the accepted norm of a society. This designation has been applied by subsequent thinkers to groups of people who have been stigmatized, marginalized, and discriminated against by virtue of, variously, their biology, origins of birth, gender, sexual identity, illness or disability, age, and income. As the public has become more conscious of the range of discrimination, the term *the other* has become more diffuse in its implications, but it always carries with it the sense of a longstanding, punitive discrimination. Foucault has also written specifically about the medical profession. In *Birth of the Clinic*, he describes how medical technologies have created a medical "gaze" that allows physicians to "see" beneath a person's skin in ways unavailable to patients. Such access has both further augmented a physician's power and contributed to the reduction of the patient to a series of mechanistic functions.

Foucault grounds his critique of medical power in its specialized knowledge, which leads to social control for its possessors. This specialized knowledge is part of the power that Howard Brody attributes to the physician in *The Healer's Power*. Brody details three kinds of power to which the physician has access: owned power, shared power, and aimed power. Owned power resides in the physician's education and his or her "acceptance of personal responsibility" for that knowledge; shared power lies in the physician's collaboration with patients in making informed decisions about their treatment; and aimed power refers to the extent to which a physician *intends* to include patients in determining their course of treatment. Brody argues that shared power offers physicians the surest way to avoid abusing their owned power or ignoring the possibility of aimed power.[3]

Howard Waitzkin defines the vulnerable position of patients in more political terms, but he also situates physicians' power in the regulatory role granted them by virtue of their specialized knowledge. Waitzkin is particularly interested in the ways that physicians do not recognize—or deliberately dismiss as irrelevant to medical care—"the big social problems" that contribute to illness.[4] Waitzkin argues that the economic forces that value production shape our ideas about social worth. Physicians stigmatize patients who cannot contribute to society in economically acceptable ways. Waitzkin cites U.S. physicians' own "upper-middle-class or corporate-class" (22) backgrounds as creating an ideological blindness that prevents them from recognizing the social contexts (poverty, gender, family/cultural traditions) that may contribute as much to patients' health as any pathology or physical dysfunction.

From Foucault, Brody, and Waitzkin, I understand power to be an interpersonal, intellectual, and social dynamic, grounded in a variety of differences among groups of people. Some of these biases are so longstanding that they are deeply buried within one's own belief system. There is, however, another element of power in medicine that is not particularly addressed by these theorists. It is grounded in the existential fear that illness, disability, or death strikes in the heart of many people—patients and physicians alike. No one can, ultimately, control death. Within this constant shadow of a power greater than anything medicine can profess to be, medical students grapple with the variety of socially based power relationships described above. How medical students learn to negotiate both their own and others' differences—and their fundamental powerlessness to defeat death—may hold the key to their ultimate comfort in being a "real doctor."

Other Patients

In a chapter titled "Thanks for Everything," Frank Vertosick Jr. recounts his miserable attempts to insert a tube from nose to stomach of a man experiencing severe nausea from an impacted bowel. Not only does his failure produce a bloody nose and more vomiting, but the patient thanks him for his efforts, only compounding the third-year student's misery:

> After almost running from the ward, I stood in the hallway to compose myself. What had just happened to this man? A total stranger had walked up to him and rammed a weapon up his nose until he was bleeding like Old Faithful, halting the torture only after he had blown lunch all over himself in full view of six other patients on the ward. On the street, this would not be called a medical procedure, but assault and battery—with witnesses, no less! And, amazingly enough, he was thankful. Thankful! For "everything."
>
> I glanced down at my white coat. This could not be ordinary clothing, I thought, it must be some sorcerer's cloak, this white linen, my only credential. It had not only shielded me from the ire of this combat veteran, but inspired his gratitude as well.
>
> In the years that followed, I would do worse things to a human body than make it puke or give it a bloody nose—a lot worse. Nevertheless, another milestone had passed. As I threw away the nasogastric tube caked

with bloody jelly, I felt the first inkling of what being a doctor involved. The intoxicant of power.

I wasn't sure I liked it. (37–38)

Vertosick interprets his situation in terms of a physician's power, power he certainly doesn't possess at the time and, in fact, is unsure he ever wants to possess. In the preceding chapters, I have quoted numerous authors regarding their discomfort with the privilege that seemed to accrue automatically to the physician, the owned power that Brody refers to and the power of specialized knowledge that Foucault describes. Vertosick's anecdote conveys a similar sense, but he adds another specific dimension. He had this experience in a Veterans Administration hospital (VA), "the Vah, or, more sarcastically, the Vah-spa—although it was hardly spa-like" (34). Because of the inefficiencies bred of bureaucracy, undergraduate medical students are given freer rein there than they might be granted elsewhere, at least in Vertosick's rotation. In this sense, veterans who are hospitalized at the VA enter a special social realm that makes them more susceptible to the hazards of being treated by physicians in training, makes them an other, different by virtue of location.

Although *all* patients, simply by being labeled as such, become an other to physicians and thus subject to a power imbalance, the abuse of medical power that is most documented has been its intentional and unintentional use against patients based on race and ethnicity, gender, sexuality, and disability.[5] In medical education, the advent of and continued debate about courses and workshops in "cultural competence" indicate that racial and other kinds of discrimination have concerned medical educators as well.[6] Such discrimination against individual patients is not described in the memoirs to the extent that it has been documented in historical and survey research. In part, I suspect, physicians who write in the first person (or their editors) are astute enough to know what is socially acceptable to say about patients. Others may be so uncomfortable with the possibility of being accused of racism that they deliberately avoid raising the issue of race at all.

Writers, however reticent about their own biases, though, are quick to criticize bias in other physicians. William Nolen condemns two surgeons who speak nonchalantly about the possibility of a child with Down syndrome surviving heart surgery: "Any doctor who could laugh about, or even take lightly, a heart operation just because the patient happened to be retarded— mongoloid [both terms in common usage at that time] children have a high incidence of congenital heart problems—was a bastard in my book. And still is" (185). Elizabeth Morgan reports her disgust with a physician's examination of a woman with appendicitis:

> Till then I had had my doubts about Dr. Chester, but now I watched him carefully. He broke into a big smile and pressed unnecessarily hard and deep, even as his patient squirmed between his hands and screamed with pain.
> "I think she's had enough, Dr. Chester," I said coldly.
> "Sorry dear. I didn't mean to hurt you." He looked at me.
> "You come over and examine her. See what a hot appendix feels like. You have to learn."
> "No thank you. She's had enough." (118–19)

Claire McCarthy suspects a greater open-mindedness toward white patients by white health professionals: "Why had nobody even mentioned AIDS in Melissa's case? . . . Was it because she was a blond little girl born to educated, upper-middle-class parents? I didn't like to think so, but maybe it was true" (181).

The memoirs do reveal, however, ways in which more subtle biases contribute to conditions that can lead to discrimination against patients. Although many writers do not mention the race or ethnicity of their patients, they often comment on the socioeconomic disadvantage that many of their patients face. J. Kenyon Rainer describes the substandard environment at the public hospital where he trained:

> The John Gaston Charity Hospital, run entirely by chief residents, was 523 beds of misery: patients suffering gunshot wounds, stab wounds, car wrecks, pneumonia, kidney failure, psychiatric disease, complicated obstetrical problems, tuberculosis, syphilis, and cancer. The patients lay in open twenty-bed wards, with no privacy except for curtains drawn on metal runners between the beds. The red brick exterior was weathered; the concrete-block wall interior, peeling and moldy. In the main walkways the checkered brown and gray linoleum floors were chipped and faded. Roaches scurried along the baseboards. The sick moaned and often turned to face the window at the end of each ward. (181)

Writers often compare the patients in public and private hospitals. "The physical differences between Bellevue patients and private paying patients," observes William Nolen, "were almost as marked as the social and sociological differences," going on to note the "omnipresen[ce]" of malnutrition and such "other complicating ailments" as tuberculosis (39–40). Robert Marion writes about "the complex social problems in the lives of many of our patients. The people who came to us for medical care were generally poor, and their poverty affected every aspect of their lives, including their health" (202). Neither of these men, however, adds that poverty undoubtedly skewed the racial composition of these patient populations.

Fitzhugh Mullan is one of the few writers who deliberately set out to grapple with the role of race in the provision of medical care. He describes the people who came to Lincoln Hospital:

> They were the people of the slum. They were not the simple peasants of some poor but integrated rural society. They were not the proud tribes-men of an emerging nation. They were the denizens of the South Bronx, escapees from the American South or American Puerto Rico, drawn lemming-like to the city, to New York. Unable to speak the language, jobless, the target of layaway plans, pimps, and hustlers of every sort, they moved into the South Bronx, where there was the highest rate of heroin addiction in the world.[7]

Most writers express compassion for patients whose poverty has placed them in circumstances detrimental to their health. When it comes to individual patients, however, they often falter. Some authors catch themselves making biased generalizations about their patients that are not simply demeaning but are medically dangerous. J. Kenyon Rainer writes about a man with alcoholism he has been seeing in the hospital for over two years, a man who had "always complained to any resident . . . that would listen." On one occasion, however, the man has a life-threatening illness whose symptoms Rainer dismisses as the patient's usual complaining. "His alcoholism had made me complacent," Rainer admits, "resulting in a critical delay in making the proper diagnosis. And now, because I had judged his character and not his disease, he was in danger of dying" (150–52).

Rainer writes about his bias against alcoholism rather than race or eth-nicity. In doing so, he is like most of these writers, who direct derogatory comments toward their patients' so-called risky behaviors. Every writer has at least one tripwire when it comes to patients. A few such examples include the following:

> Mrs. Hammerman was back in again. . . . She's a woman with hypertension who periodically drinks herself into a stupor and has to be brought in to be nursed along until she wakes up. I decided that Mrs. Hammerman could

just drop dead as far as I was concerned, and I stuck to my guns for a while, but after blinking at the ceiling for a half-hour and getting myself so mad I couldn't sleep, I tossed in the towel and went up to see the woman.[8]

If "Tijuana Special" has a callous ring to it, the term [for an illegal abortion] was, nonetheless, an accurate reflection of our attitudes towards the women who had them. First of all, we considered them a real pain; they kept the resident on duty up half the night. . . . We had contempt for these women, who, we thought, had been stupid or irresponsible about birth control.[9]

That I had these feelings doesn't mean that I didn't hate junkies. Junkies were among the most manipulative, venal, outrightly criminal, and narcissistic of all the patients I ever dealt with. A junkie is destructive of himself and everyone around him and will engage in such destructive behavior over and over and over until he is dead or until he has quit.[10]

"If you don't admit me," [Mollie] said slowly and deliberately, "I'll go home and kill my son and myself with gas."

There was a long pause. Jerry excused himself, and we left the room. He was furious. "She has got us by the balls. She knows the system better than I do. I can't turn away a suicide or homicide threat. It's too big a risk."

. . . Mollie was sitting alone in the little side room, smoking a cigarette. After I told her that her son had arrived, she smiled faintly but made no move to go to him. I went back to the little boy and asked him if he wanted to visit his mother. He looked solemnly at me and said simply, "No." I felt overwhelming sadness for him and all the lousy breaks he was getting. . . . I wanted to feel sympathy for [his mother], but I hated her because of what she was doing to her son.[11]

Although race or ethnicity is not mentioned here, readers can still infer that many of these patients, seen in public institutions and given the country's socioeconomic demographics, are very likely people of color. The tendency of writers to generalize to all of their patients runs the danger of seeing race or ethnicity when the real problem may lie in poverty and lack of access to adequate health care or education.

Some writers express a particular fondness for patients that most of the world has given up on. For example, Emily Transue writes, "Despite occasional sparring on both sides—a new resident with a bad attitude toward these dirty and needy and down-and-out patients, a patient getting violent in the throes of intoxication or withdrawal—the relationship overall between the ER staff and the alcoholics is a remarkably cordial one. I sense affection on both sides" (194). The deliberately satiric tone that characterizes much of Joseph Sacco's prose often masks genuine concern for his patients: "Junkies are virtually wholly dependent on the kindness of strangers to rescue them from their dilemma [of being at high risk for HIV infection]. And, for the vast majority, strangers have not been very kind. Such shabby treatment is a pity, a damn shame, because not only does it reflect the callousness of society, but it is the major factor that puts society at risk for the further spread of AIDS" (75). Waitzkin assumes that most people who choose medicine as a career desire to help others, but their education, which does not prepare physicians to address the social ills that contribute to their patients' ill health, renders them unequipped to handle such dilemmas.[12] On the whole, these memoirs show young physicians painfully aware of the inadequacies of medicine to treat all that is wrong with their patients. They struggle to maintain their generosity, some with greater success than others, in situations where they are doomed to fail.

In general, memoirists of recent years seem to express more acceptance of patients' so-called risky behaviors than do writers of memoirs published before about 1985. Toward one behavior, however, memoirists over the years have shown unremitting scorn: overeating. Although being over- or underweight can be a factor in some medical conditions, some writers' comments about weight are gratuitous, extending to people who are not even their patients. J. Kenyon Rainer remarks, "I punched the buzzer on the outside steel door, and about five minutes later a heavy nurse waddled to the door" (188). Observations of a patient's weight sometimes serve only to denigrate the patient: "Obese and comatose, she was difficult to ignore," notes Stephen A. Hoffmann (90). Of a patient being checked the day after "a gastric bypass operation for severe obesity," Craig A. Miller remarks, "As the corpulent Mrs. B shakes her head, we file out of her room" (17). From Dr. X: "I went in and saw her. God, what a repulsive creature. She weighed about 250 pounds and had a huge filthy gauze pad stuck down across her belly to cover a big draining sore" (197). Claire McCarthy remarks on the size of nearly every person who might be considered overweight, often in connection with other disparaging observations: "The woman in the corner holding the baby was heavy. . . . She had curly black hair that needed washing, and her red-and-white checked dress was way too big for her" (156).

More than direct expressions of cultural bias, memoirs of medical education contain examples of what has come to be called blaming the victim, seen here as a simple lack of compassion for the circumstances that have brought someone to a hospital bed. As Ron Maggiore describes to the readers of his blog the eight patients he admitted one day his posting vacillates between compassion and frustration as he tries to be nonjudgmental but ultimately succumbs to blame: "You see a common theme in the majority of patients admitted to the U for medicine, but I try to look past it, help them out, but I don't forget the fact that she [an obese, asthmatic, diabetic woman] had pretty much set herself up for this horrible exacerbation."[13] At their most cynical—perhaps because speakers so seldom hear the blame they speak—professionals hold dying patients to blame for the fatal events of their illnesses. Emily Transue identifies the practice in the language of cardiac arrest:

> In reference to a patient, "to code" means to die, to have a cardiac or pulmonary arrest. "It was almost the end of the surgery and suddenly he just coded." At first this phrasing seemed strange to me. It sounded as if people did it on purpose, the way we say "She failed chemotherapy" as though it were a character flaw. Soon the phrase became familiar and ceased to bother me. (43)

This kind of language can be applied to patients who may be very similar, culturally, to the speakers. Thus, as I noted at the beginning of this chapter, the very notion of *patienthood* becomes a marker of difference through which power falls directly into the physician's hands.

Other Physicians

As Waitzkin and others have pointed out, the people admitted to U.S. medical schools well into the mid-1900s were predominately white, male, Protestant, and presumed heterosexual and not disabled. At one point, quota systems actually maintained this status quo, but those systems eventually disappeared during the 1960s, in the face of the rise of equal opportunity in education.[14] The 1960s also saw a rise in the number of women and African Americans (both men and women) applying to predominately white medical schools. Men's memoirs of medical education begin to mention women as classmates by the mid-1980s; references to African American or Hispanic students or residents also appear, but much less frequently.

The memoirs that I am examining do not lend themselves to extensive analysis of many of the so-called underrepresented groups of students in medical school. From African American physicians, I have found only *How to Survive Medical School* by Toni Martin, a mixture of practical advice and personal anecdote, in which Martin identifies herself briefly as African American; the memoirs of Ben Carson (*Gifted Hands* and *The Big Picture*), an internationally famous neurosurgeon who has written mostly about his career and his faith; and *Forged by the Knife*, by surgeon Patricia L. Dawson, a series of extensive interviews with other African American women surgeons. None of these works matches exactly my criteria of book-length, education-focused memoirs. Nor do Rafael Campo's essays about medical education and practice, in which he identifies himself as Cuban American, gay, and a poet; Lisa Iezzoni's study of mobility, which includes the story of her diagnosis with multiple sclerosis while a medical student; Abraham Verghese's book in which his South Asian identity is a part of his interaction with his community; Lori Arviso Alvord's account of her work as a Navajo woman surgeon, with a chapter about her medical education and residency; Cuban American Pedro José Greer's book about providing healthcare to the homeless of Miami, also with a chapter about his medical education; or Kevin M. Takakuwa, Nick Rubashkin, and Karen E. Herzig's edited collection of essays by medical students who identify themselves as culturally different from their classmates.

This disparity, however, reflects the rate and number in which other "underrepresented" groups have entered medical school. The emergence of women's memoirs parallels the increase of women in medicine, a numerical parallel that has not yet occurred for different racial groups. Of the forty or so memoirs I have used for this study, fifteen are by women, still a small number but one about which I feel more comfortable generalizing than for any other designated minority group in medical schools. Sayantani DasGupta writes from a feminist rather than a race perspective in *Her Own Medicine: A Woman's Journey from Student to Doctor*. In *What Patients Taught Me* Audrey Young makes one observation about the awkwardness of being Asian in rural Montana but no observations about feeling uncomfortable as a female student or resident. Gender is discussed by women in three general ways: reports of overtly sexist behaviors by men; reflections on what it means to be a woman physician; and descriptions, usually not cast in terms of gender, that reveal a gender*ed* ethos underlying medical practice and education.

The history of women in medicine has been widely studied and eloquently documented.[15] For my purposes, I note simply that the entrance of large numbers of women into medicine in the last quarter of the twentieth century parallels a similar movement a century earlier. Both periods were marked by a rising desire among women for professional work in general, and medical work in particular, a dissatisfaction with many of the methods and manners in which medicine was being practiced (by men), and a social climate ready to push for greater opportunities for women. Even so, the acceptance of women into medical schools in significant numbers met with resistance. Nevertheless, by 1923 women comprised 6 percent of the enrollment in medical schools, a triumph in the eyes of those who had fought, one at a time, for the admission of women. (This percentage reflects admission only to "regular" medical schools, that is, those teaching the philosophies and practices of allopathic medicine rather than "irregular" practices such as homeopathy, hydropathy, etc.)[16] They believed that their war was won. Such, however, was not the case. By 1940, only 5 percent of graduates of medical schools were women; in 1960 (notwithstanding a brief doubling of enrollment toward the end of World War II) that percentage stood at only 5.7. In 1965, female graduates of medical schools rose by 1.1 percent, to 6.8 percent, the largest increase in nearly thirty years.[17] Even so, enrollment had remained relatively unchanged for over forty years.

Since 1965, however, and unlike the decrease of women entering medicine after the initial breakthrough in the early 1900s, the number of women entering medical schools has steadily continued to rise. From 6.8 percent of graduating students in 1965, by 1975 graduation of women reached 13.4 percent, nearly double.[18] Fifteen years later, in 1990, the percentage had again more than doubled, reaching 33.9 percent, then up to 42.6 percent in 1999, and 45.9 percent in 2004.[19] By way of comparison, in 1965, when women comprised 6.8 percent of the graduates nationwide, that number was surpassed by the total enrollment of students of color, at 10.7 percent. By 1975, however, women graduates were over twice that of students of color: 13.4 percent as opposed to 6.3 percent. In 1999, with 42.6 percent of graduating students women (including women of color), only 15.2 percent were members of "underrepresented minority groups," of which African American students comprised 7.7 percent.[20] (At some point in their counting, the American Medical Association separated ethnicities, with a special category for Asian/Pacific Islander, a group I am not including in my report of students of color and which the AMA does not include as an underrepresented minority group.)

The steady increase in memoirs of medical education by women reflects this growth of women in medical schools. These memoirs fall into three distinct clusters. The first cluster, published between 1976 and 1983 (covering undergraduate and graduate medical education from about 1963 through 1978) includes at least six books: *Woman Doctor* by Florence Haseltine and Yvonne Yaw; *The Cutting Edge* by Joni Lynn Scalia; *The Making of a Woman Surgeon* by Elizabeth Morgan; *A Woman in Residence* by Michelle Harrison; *Woman/Doctor* by Jane Patterson and Lynda Madaras; and *How to Survive Medical School* by Toni Martin. The middle four of these are memoirs, the last a quasi-memoir (as I described earlier), and the first a "documentary with fictional elements," whose depiction of "the sex bias and its manifestations are real."[21] (I have not included Haseltine's accounts in my study.) Four of the writers (Haseltine, Morgan, Harrison, and Patterson) wrote with the explicit purpose of critiquing the medical profession's treatment of women physicians as well as women patients. Three of these writers—Haseltine, Harrison, and Patterson—were, by the time they published their stories, leaders in the emerging women's health movement.

All these writers describe overt sexism throughout the course of their education. They write at length about their interviews for medical school or residency. Jane Patterson's account is typical:

> At one school I was interviewed by a panel of doctors. . . .
>
> Most of their questions ran along the lines of, "Did I have a boyfriend?" "Was I engaged?" "Did I plan to get married and have children?" . . . It would never have occurred to me to challenge my interviewers' right to ask these questions. All I was concerned about was getting the right answers, which I was beginning to realize might be rather tricky. I wanted to sound like a normal, feminine female, but I also wanted to let them know that I was serious about a career and that my career came first. (76–77)

Once in medicine, the women often face confrontations like the one reported by Joni Lynn Scalia from the vice director of radiology, where she was serving a residency: "I don't like women; I don't think they belong in medicine, and I particularly don't think they belong in radiology" (137). Toni Martin speculates that gender was a harder bias to overcome than race in the 1970s, as she observed how she and her husband, also in medical school and also African American, were treated by the same teachers:

> On any written test, I would do as well or better than he, including the tests we took at the end of every clerkship. I also tended to talk more in classes, asking questions or offering answers. However, I was repeatedly criticized

for being too quiet. It was obvious to both of us that no one was going to call a six-feet, three-inch black man nonassertive, even if he never opened his mouth. On the only clerkship we took on the same ward at the same time, he was recommended for honors but placed too low on the written test to receive them, whereas I, who received the second highest grade out of a class of 150 students, was not recommended for honors because I failed to make a strong enough impression. It is said that doctors like to create doctors in their own image, so the further you deviate from that image, the harder it is going to be. And my experience suggests that the opposite sex is perceived as more deviant than another race. (71–72)

Most of the women do not entertain the idea of marrying or having children during their training. Michelle Harrison reports receiving little advice from older women physicians, who were uncomfortable even talking about motherhood. They either spoke of children as an imposition or in whispers. "Have your children early and get it over with [so that when] you are practicing, you don't have to bother with little children," one woman advises, and another talks about her family as if "children were not a fit topic of conversation" (67).

Female writers from this period all report sexist behavior by male colleagues, peers as well as professors: off-color jokes derogatory of women in both social and work settings; slides of female breasts in anatomy lectures; direct statements about the inappropriateness of women in medicine. All of them encounter quandaries about appearance and propriety. Should I wear my hair long or short? styled or pulled back? Should I wear a dress or the ill-fitting surgical scrubs (pants and shirts that, in the earlier years of women's entry into medical schools, were cut only in men's sizes)? Do I sleep in the call room with the men? and if I do, do I keep my clothes on? Do I change for surgery in the doctors'—men's—dressing room? or do I change with the nurses—women—in a different area? And why aren't there more restrooms for women? As late as 1997, student Michael Greger notes in his journal, "The bathrooms in the hospital are segregated. There are bathrooms marked 'Patients' and bathrooms marked 'Nurses.' Worse—the two OR locker rooms; one's marked 'Doctors' and the other is marked 'Women'" (11).

All of the women writers from this period note, with sorrow, the lack of women on the faculty who could serve as models for them. The few women they encounter often seem like caricatures of the worst stereotypes of the cold, overachieving, unsympathetic woman doctor. Elizabeth Morgan writes,

"There were very few women doctors at Yale, or anywhere, and they were intelligent, efficient and severe in looks and manner. My dream then was to become as sharp, cool and commanding as they were. It took me many years to learn that their manner—and their overtly critical attitude toward women medical students—reflected their insecurity and jealous protection of their own uncertain position in a man's world" (67). Even with the increase of women in medicine over the intervening forty years, their numbers are still uncommonly low in academic medicine,[22] and many women writers of recent years voice the same complaints. Emily Baldwin says: "'How old is too old to have kids?' we ask all the time. . . . Despite the fact that there are many, many women in medicine these days, I have yet to find anyone I can look at as a role model in this area."[23]

Women meet the more superficial evidence of medicine's unpreparedness for women physicians with varying degrees of humor and frustration, but they always write seriously about seeking to enter a profession that is often openly hostile to their presence. When Jane Patterson struggles to hide her grief for dying patients, she gives these emotions a female identity, the Lady:

> I'd vowed to be as tough, as unemotional, as professional, as any of my male colleagues. And on the outside I was. No one ever saw me cry. But on the inside it was another story. They were, of course, entirely right about women doctors. I knew, because I knew how it was inside me.
>
> Inside me there was a lone woman in long robes, standing at the edge of a darkened lake, wringing her hands in sorrow and weeping in despair. The Lady never did anything. She just stood there crying. I had no use for her and would like to have been rid of her. (14)

Patterson's memoir, in fact, turns in large part upon her coming to accept—and liberate—this Lady, who is also lesbian. Elizabeth Morgan recounts a familiar version of the "damned if you do, damned if you don't" scenario reported by most of the writers in this first cluster. As a second-year resident who has carefully disciplined herself to match her male peers in every task, Morgan is upset when a female intern, Patsy, tries to lighten her workload by asking others to do her work. When Morgan reprimands her for this unprofessional behavior, Morgan herself is taken to task by the other (male) residents and, more important, by her supervising physician, Dr. Mulvaney. She reports the following conversation with her mother:

"You won't be fired, I'm certain, but you might stop and think about yourself. Being a woman in surgery is much harder than you like to admit. Patsy has adapted by not fighting, and letting men feel sorry for her. It makes a lot of men feel noble and grand and protective. You've adapted by making things as hard for yourself as possible. Now you're being seen as a hard woman who won't even help out another woman. Do you want to be seen that way?"

"No, of course not. I'm *not* that way."

"Then from now till the end of your residency, don't criticize anyone and don't fight with anyone. Apologize to Dr. Mulvaney, and offer to do the work Patsy won't do herself."

"Oh, God. But Mark [another intern] wouldn't do the work either, and he's not in trouble."

"He's not a woman. Don't you see, Patsy's turned many of the men against you. She behaves the way they expect a woman to behave, so when you demand that she behave like any other surgeon, as you do, they take her side." She sighed. "I'm afraid surgical residency hasn't been good for you *or* Patsy." (287)

In these two passages, Patterson and Morgan struggle to sort out what kind of woman, physician, and *woman physician* they want to be. In doing so, they must consider to what extent their public face has been shaped by the eyes and minds of the men who surround them.

The second cluster of memoirs by women covers the years 1984-1995 but includes only three books by two authors: Dorothy Greenbaum and Deidre S. Laiken's *Lovestrong: A Woman Doctor's True Story of Marriage and Medicine* and Perri Klass's *A Not Entirely Benign Procedure: Four Years as a Medical Student* and *Baby Doctor: A Pediatrician's Training*. Both writers note many of the same kinds of bias reported in the earlier memoirs, but discrimination against women in medicine is not a primary focus for these books. Of the two, Klass brings a more deliberately feminist perspective to some of her experiences, which often turn on notions of identity more nuanced than those written by women in the first cluster. For example, in her essay "Baby Poop" Klass ponders her medical team's response when she offers to change the obviously dirty diaper of a newborn baby.

At first, she speculates that "the doctors were squeamish about seeing a diaper changed," perhaps being childless themselves. Then, she told herself, it was really about "dignity. *Doctors don't change diapers*" (Klass's italics). Next, she offers a feminist analysis about changing diapers as women's work. In the hospital, then, "the diaper was changed by a nurse, a woman doing a woman's job." In the end, however, Klass concludes that the answer is more complex and reflects her own development as a physician:

> But when I thought further about [it] . . . it occurred to me that in fact my willingness to change the baby's diaper had something to do with my own attitudes toward the sexual politics of medicine. A year earlier, I'm not sure I would have offered. When I first started out in the hospital, I wouldn't have offered, simply because I never offered to do anything unless I was sure it was my place. If none of the doctors had mentioned it, I wouldn't have either; I would have been worried that perhaps my diaper-changing technique was not smooth enough to show off in front of an attending. And then, after I got over those first-time jitters, I went through a period in which I was very sensitive about sexism. I worried that if I did anything that marked me too distinctly as female, I would be respected less. I resented being mistaken for a nurse. I didn't talk much about my own child. . . .
>
> But I got over most of this nonsense. By the time I met the baby in my story, I think I had honestly come to believe that both my experiences as a woman and my special skills as a parent add something to my abilities as a doctor. . . . I offered to [change the diaper] because I knew I could do it and I wanted the baby to be wearing a clean diaper. And if anyone had made any cracks about female doctors, I would have despised him, and not myself.[24]

Klass regales a friend of hers, a woman who is not a physician, with this analysis, after which the friend asks only one question: "Was the baby okay?" Chagrined, Klass concludes, "What can I say? Isn't that obviously the right question to ask? Isn't that the detail I completely omitted from my story? . . . And when I was congratulating myself on my ability to escape the doctor's perspective, just because I offered to change the diaper, I was in fact as caught up in my own performance as any of those doctors" (166). Klass broadens her feminist critique of both her own and others' possible responses to Klass as a woman and a mother, going on to describe a socialization process that overrides gender.

From the ten years 1996 to 2005, I have discovered nine memoirs (seven books and two blogs) about medical education or residency by women. Only one of them, *Her Own Medicine* by Sayantani DasGupta, makes a feminist critique central to her writing. Although most of the writers note some overt sexism and think occasionally about what it means to them to be a woman in medicine, some of them do not consider gender at all. Does this mean that sexism has disappeared from medical education? Less overt commentary or behavior is reported in the later memoirs than in the earlier ones, but men may simply be more legally and politically savvy than in the past—and some women more adept at parrying barbs or choosing which battles to fight. Women are also finding a larger community of women among their classmates. Where earlier writers often remarked upon seeking out the two or three other women in their class but often finding little ground for friendship, authors in this last cluster write without comment about friendships with both women and men. Marriage and childbirth occur, often written about for the romance and excitement of it all, not about its uniqueness in the setting of medical education. Still, studies from medical schools across the country regularly attest to the ongoing harassment of women medical students.[25]

At this point it becomes instructive to examine these women's memoirs alongside those of their male peers. Although the men write with concern about being a responsible partner or parent while in medical school or residency, they never define those problems as direct products of being men. When they encounter animosity from teachers or peers, they do not wonder whether it is because they are men. When men and women write about the things that trouble them the most about medical education, however, the similarities in their complaints can be cast in a broader discussion of gender. Take the following three issues:

DESTRUCTION OF HUMAN SPIRIT   In earlier chapters, I described students' and residents' fears of a loss of self, in the sense of a whole human being who inhabits a world and an emotional range broader than medicine. Emily Transue describes her years of residency in terms of a sad narrowing of her sensibility:

> After I finished residency, counting was one of the hardest things to unlearn. It took an existential shift to cease envisioning my life in terms of blocks to be checked off, days to be gotten through. Ironically, residency taught me to see life as a precious and tenuous thing, one that could be snatched from anyone at any moment. Yet it put me in the habit of

treating my own life like an obstacle course, a series of unpleasant tasks to be raced through as quickly as possible, as if it was the end and not the process that was important.

People have asked, at the time and since, whether I liked residency. The question baffles me as much now as it did then. Am I glad I did it? Yes. I never learned so much or grew as much in any three years, and never will. Would I do it again? No. I can't conceive of mustering that kind of energy again. Once in a lifetime was enough. Was it pleasant? No, on the whole, though moments were. It was satisfying, sometimes fun, but never easy.

Was it horrible? No. Still, by the third year I was counting hours, and at the end I counted minutes. (199)

Craig A. Miller is even blunter: "While it's true that the residency programs produce excellent surgeons, there still must be some alternative to a system that chews up individuals and crushes families with such ruthless efficiency. We must be able to train surgeons without destroying their lives" (238). Transue and Miller describe the creation of competent, even compassionate physicians who are, nevertheless, automatons because they have been forced to deny the personal side of their lives.

FEARS OF WEAKNESS   Patterson is not alone in hiding her emotions from both her colleagues and herself. Writers across the years record instances when they feel too emotionally overwhelmed to do their work, often with a secret dread that they will never be able to live up to others' image of the cool-headed, in-control physician. Providing emergency treatment to a patient at a time when she is also grieving for the recent death of a dear friend, Danielle Ofri writes, "I felt too young and too small to carry this burden. If this was what it meant to be a doctor—to allow my patient to collapse the weight of his fears against me, while juggling my own pains . . .—I didn't think I was strong enough. I wasn't sure if I would ever be strong enough" (111). Stephen A. Hoffmann describes his emotional withdrawal from patients as a deliberate strategy to avoid the feelings he faced during his time working in the intensive care unit (ICU):

Wavering constantly between hope and despair during my stay in the ICU, I often had the feeling that some greater force was at work with my feelings, whimsically and deliberately playing with them.

As a result, I found it more and more risky to extend myself emotionally to my patients, more and more threatening to get close to them. I grew cautious about allowing myself to be drawn into their lives at all, even going so far as to keep patients at arm's length. It was simply too hard to grow attached to them and to see them hurt. (100)

In these passages, Ofri and Hoffmann grapple with finding a way to manage the emotional upheaval that accompanies much of their work. Hoffmann finds himself withholding emotional attachment, while Ofri feels that she cannot shoulder the weight that a patient's physical and emotional need places on her.

DEVALUATION OF CARING   Even if students and young physicians feel that they can manage their emotions, they often believe that these emotions are deemed inappropriate in a physician. Men and women alike report being criticized, by both male and female residents and attendings, for being too soft. When they *do* encounter physicians who condone this more personal kind of caring, they report these conversations at some length. Intern Emily Transue, upset by the impending death of one of her patients, is comforted by a female resident who tells of a similar experience:

> "I went back to the residents' room, and I just lost it. The rest of the team came in and I was there, sobbing, and they were like, what, what? And I told them, and you know what they said? They said: 'If you're that thin-skinned, if you're going to let things get to you like that, you shouldn't be in medicine.'
>
> "That's what they said. And I spun on them and I said: 'If I ever stop letting things get to me, that's when I'll quit medicine.'
>
> "And it turned out the chief resident of psychiatry was sitting there, listening to all this—I hadn't even seen him—and he stood and said, 'That's the sanest thing I've heard all week.'"
>
> I smile through the tears that are rolling down my cheeks again.
>
> "It's not a bad thing to cry, okay? More than that: it's the right thing. It's what you need to do—for yourself, and for your patients, too. Don't give that up, okay? Don't let anybody talk you out of it."
>
> I nod.
>
> "Sit here for a bit, if you need to, all right?" (108–09)

Robert Marion writes about a time during his third year of undergraduate medical education when he was sent to oversee the reception of a child who had been brought, dead, to the emergency room:

So I stood, alone in the ambulance port, crying inconsolably on that hot August morning.

After a few minutes Lynn [the ER nurse] came out to find me. . . . Seeing the state I was in, she put her arm around my shoulder and gently . . . led me to the now empty isolation room and called Mark [the resident] over, stat. The resident immediately left his patient, saying as he entered the room, "This better be important." After taking one look at me sitting in a chair, holding my head in my hands, and sobbing softly to myself, he asked, "What happened, Bob?"

When I couldn't answer, Lynn spoke, "I sent him out to declare a SIDS and I found him like this out in the ambulance port."

"Your first dead baby?" Mark asked. I nodded. "I remember mine," he said, flopping down on the other chair in the room. "A kid who fell out of a fifth-story window during the summer of my internship. It's funny; he barely had a scratch on him. He looked fine, except for the fact that he was stone dead. I felt horrible. I had nightmares about him for months. I'm sorry it had to happen to you."

I had calmed down a little by then. Mark and Lynn stayed with me as long as they could, but a little before nine they were called out for an emergency. . . . I remained in the isolation room for nearly two hours. At about ten-thirty, when I felt I could once again cope with life, I stepped out of the room into an ER buzzing with activity. (48–49)

The residents in these two instances affirm the emotions of their charges. They also acknowledge having the same feelings—and are not ashamed to admit it. They take time to talk to Transue and Marion, in the latter case dropping a tone of impatience ("This better be important") upon understanding the situation, and allow their charges to spend some time alone before going back into the flurry of hospital work.

The situations that physicians in training often find the most emotionally distressing involve a loss of balance or wholeness in their lives, isolation from peers, and a denigration of caring emotions. Moreover, students and residents feel they must hide feelings of grief and self-doubt from others—sometimes even from themselves. The qualities of connection, caring, and emotional openness run counter to an educational and professional ethos that values independence, distance, and objectivity. Although these latter three qualities are also important, even necessary at times, for a physician to perform in situations of physical and emotional pressure, without the former qualities as counterbalance they can solidify into rigid dogmatism, cynicism, or condescension.

The first three qualities have traditionally been attributed to women, the second three to men. Although it is intellectually dangerous to link behaviors or emotional proclivities directly to sex chromosomes, circumstances of history and sexual politics *have* tended to connect feelings of caring and connection with women and independence and self-assertion with men.[26] In the introduction to this study, I speculated that a national identity that overemphasizes independence and vaunts larger-than-life deeds may have helped create an image of the heroic physician that is as one-sided as it is inaccurate. Given that the American hero was also, almost always, a man, it is not surprising that the popular image of the American Doctor misrepresents all physicians and is doubly uncomfortable for many women.

Generalizing about the experience of other minority groups of medical students or residents from the experience of women should be done with extreme caution. It is hardly a new observation, however, that any person deemed to be some kind of cultural other will find medical school even more difficult than it already is. The dangers of isolation and self-doubt that plague all students will take on an added dimension. The gendered tradition of medical education and practice, moreover, prompts a consideration of how other groups' cultural values might be similarly disavowed or simply ignored. People from cultures that favor connection and deference over hierarchy and autonomy, for example, or people with disabilities such that they do not communicate primarily by verbal or written U.S. speech, may discover themselves uncomfortable with the traditional male model of the U.S. physician.

Other Students

Discussions of power, oppression, and the other in medicine place the physician, whatever his or her other cultural identities, at the pinnacle of power over patients. Medical students, as future physicians and by the advantages that have brought most of them to medical school, also hold a privileged position in relation to the patients they will see. From the minute they are accepted into medical school, however, students enter a liminal space in which they are seen as both a physician and not a physician. With such uncertain status, and falling under the scrutiny of countless groups of people (patients, teachers, family), medical students may come to see themselves, with discomfort and confusion, as the other in a variety of situations.

When Danielle Ofri's grandfather was dying, her family turned to her as their spokesperson. "My family allowed me, without argument," she writes, "to assume the role of medical emissary for them. But I was only a first-year medical student then, and my family couldn't have known how little I knew" (11). Such flattery sometimes pleases students, but just as often the premature designation makes them uncomfortable. When Melvin Konner and his wife were asked about their experience with midwives, he writes, "I tried to distinguish between what I might say as a doctor (or medical student) and what I might say as a father," and he realizes that his "lay status was gone forever. . . . A suggestion from me was now a suggestion from a medically trained person. It carried legal as well as moral responsibility" (250, 252).

Conversely, medical students often discover that friends and family have limits to what they want to hear about medicine. For example, Perri Klass has to be reminded at one point "that [friends] find [dissecting dogs] an inappropriate topic for dinner-table conversation. I am becoming a bore, I think."[27] Some students and residents find themselves reluctant to talk about what they've seen, either to protect the person they're talking to or to avoid having to talk about something that they fear will upset a loved one. J. Kenyon Rainer writes, "Julie [his wife] always asked about my day, but I remained vague. There was no remedy in reliving the death of a patient; no compliment necessary for saving a life" (119).

Students and residents learn that some things can be spoken about only among peers, but they also report that there are things they feel they can't say to other students or residents. These often concern feelings of inadequacy or sorrow. Claire McCarthy remembers feeling as if she were the only student bothered by dissection: "I was upset and full of the knowledge that this cadaver was the body of a real person—but I was too embarrassed to say anything, too embarrassed to ask to leave. I searched the other faces in the room, trying to find some sign that someone was feeling the same way, but I could find nothing. Already we were learning to hide how we felt. I probably didn't show anything on my face, either" (6). Steve Horowitz offers an example of how expressions of grief were closed off in his residency:

> A surgical resident I knew had a way of dealing with death, particularly those that were tragic.
>
> "Fuck him if he can't take a joke," the resident used to say about the dead patient.

You have to try to harden yourself against death. Sometimes you laugh. You don't want to go through the rest of your life always seeing Jesse Jefferson's face in your dreams. Or remembering Anna Wilson's empty bed. So you believe you're hard and joke about writing an order to tell the patient to put his head between his legs so he can kiss his ass good-bye. (161)

Anger and gallows humor are generally accepted forms of expression among undergraduate and graduate medical students, as is an expected level of anxiety about passing exams or clerkships, but expressions of serious self-doubt or grief are usually kept private or shared with only a trusted few.

The vocal, often jocular camaraderie of medical students and residents hides—or prevents others from voicing—feelings that keep many people on emotional tenterhooks at various times throughout their medical education. So does a style of clinical teaching called *pimping*, in which questions are asked in an almost baiting manner. Although some writers find that this aggressive technique (not used as much now as in the past, it seems, but still a recurring source of complaint) is a good teaching method, more people respond with anxiety and inner fury.[28] Kenneth Klein writes, "Twice a week the other student and I have to present cases to the visit. One of the visit's functions, I'm told, is to make students twist and squirm in front of the entire ward team. This somehow enhances learning" (152). Frank Huyler criticizes an attending physician for her harsh treatment of one of the softer-spoken students: "I felt sorry for him—it seemed harsh, cruel, and we were all struggling. It was a world of superficial impressions, where an authoritative tone and firm demeanor went far, and most of us learned to be actors on rounds. Tony didn't get it, though" (28). Michael J. Collins questions the same pedagogical reasoning at the residency level: "Embarrassing the junior resident is considered a good thing. It is supposed to encourage him to study harder" (7). Whatever its success, pimping is a pedagogical method designed to impress upon its recipient the power of the person in control of the questions.

Both men and women write about crying during their hours in the hospital. In the two passages quoted in the previous section, Emily Transue and Robert Marion write about the tears that accompanied their grief for patients. Memoirists also report less-altruistic causes for tears. Stephen A. Hoffmann describes his tears as a response to "the disparity between my expectations and my ability" (53). Perri Klass writes about crying after a long and difficult night in the hospital. I had gotten only two hours of sleep, and toward morning, a young patient had died of cancer. I was sitting in the nurses' coffee room, staring into space, when the intern, who had had no sleep at all, who had been responsible for everything on the ward, came in and found me.

"Are you okay," he asked, and I promptly burst into tears.

And then I lied. I told the intern that I was crying for . . . the patient, and for her parents, but I knew that in large part I was crying for myself. I was crying because I hadn't slept much, and because I had a long day in front of me in which I would be put on the spot and have my ignorance revealed again and again.[29]

Klass states very clearly that self-pity played a large role in her distress. It crops up in nearly all the memoirs, in moments of stress or tiredness or simple impatience. Danielle Ofri grumbles, "But here we were just in a dull operation, chasing down a uterus for reasons that no one had bothered to tell me. In the haze of my mind there was a vague reminder to my body that, according to its biorhythms, it should be asleep. If this were a regular delivery I could convince my body that it was worth it" (41). The feeling extends into residency, as Michael J. Collins notes: "Sometimes it seemed there was so much bullshit. Patients could be rude to us and we had to take it. Attendings could abuse us and we had to take it. Silly, senseless jobs that had nothing to do with our education needed doing and we had to do them. . . . We had to live with all the ambiguities of being thirty-year-old highly educated men and still in positions of subservience" (219). Inherent in many of these complaints is the sense of being disregarded and mistreated. The tired student or resident has become, in his or her own eyes, an other, a powerless pawn in a limbo of never-ending demands and demeaning work. The possibility of ever ascending to power equal to one's attending physician, for no other purpose than finally to escape being ordered around, is beyond most sufferers' ability to imagine.

Students or residents who perceive themselves as other to their teachers often find it a short step to viewing themselves as other to their patients as well. In his diary, John MacNab is able to recognize the illogic in his anger with a patient, but his bitterness still echoes in his writing:

I went this afternoon to visit my real Slum Goddess, the Public Health patient with whom I had to set up an appointment. The slum she lived in was in a part of the city diametrically opposed to my own—20 miles there and 20 miles back.

That makes 40 miles.

She wasn't in. They didn't know when to expect her.

I was furious. Nobody does that to me. (She did.)

Later, I figure out that she had a perfect right to miss our appointment.

There was nothing in it for her. (158)

Stephen A. Hoffmann writes, "If, for example, an intoxicated man came in with chest pain just when I had planned to go to bed, I would mutter to myself, 'If it hadn't been for you I could have gone to sleep'" (180).

In these instances, patients are perceived as willful and inconsiderate, but students and residents often go on to imagine that patients are deliberately punishing them. As illogical as this may be (although some students' or physicians' behaviors may merit some punishment), this perception sees the more politically powerless other—the patient, often in extremis—as more powerful than the healthy person ineptly inserting needles into veins or pounding on a silent chest. "Never, never, never let them make you cry," Joseph Sacco says of his patients on Cloud Pavillion. "And, if they did make you cry, never let 'em see you do it. Don't give them the satisfaction" (28). Philip Reilly writes of seeing his patient, Mr. Grupp, "an ancient, emaciated, nearly comatose man" dying of pneumonia, as "part of the plot to deprive me of sleep" (226). Danielle Ofri writes about allowing her rage to attribute malicious motives to a patient who rudely refused treatment: "I hated him for embarrassing me in front of Sarita. I hated him for knowing that 'watchful waiting' had been a cop-out on my part. . . . I hated him for knowing just how terrified I was at the responsibility of being a doctor" (122).

The irrationality of these students' and residents' reasoning only underscores the extent of the alienation they are feeling. Nearly all of the memoirsts write about moments like this, not proudly, but with a sad recognition of the unworthiness of their response. So horrifying is this reversal of perspective on power that Robert Marion uses it as the primary image to measure the depth of his moral descent during his residency. Early in his memoir, pointedly titled *Learning to Play God*, he describes his horror as an intern repeatedly stabs a severely ill woman in unsuccessful attempts to draw blood late at night. Marion watches as the intern rails, "Just what I said: she should be dead. This woman has multisystem failure. . . . There's no way anybody can do anything to fix her. . . . If she'd had the decency to die last weekend like she should have I'd be in bed now, sound asleep; instead she lived, so

I've got to keep trying to get blood out of her for this stupid sepsis workup."
When he protests at the intern's cruelty, Marion writes, "Al glared at me
and shook his head. 'You don't understand, do you?' he said. 'You just don't
understand'" (28).

As Marion leaves the hospital that night he promises himself to "never
allow myself to think about a patient [that] way" (29), but less than two years
later, two months into his own internship, he relates his own dark night on
call, faced in an intensive care unit with a newborn baby whose intravenous
line has fallen out once again. The baby is soon crying, with bleeding and
bruises at several sites on his body. The nurse, Barbara, suggests that Marion
stop, at first gently but with increasing urgency, until, finally,

> Barbara stood by watching me, horrified as I jabbed the baby's leg over
> and over again, until at last she commanded, "Bob, enough is enough!
> Take out that needle right now, and call the resident!"
>
> I stopped and stared at her; my eyes were burning, my scrub suit was
> soaked, and the insides of my sneakers were damp with perspiration. I had
> been working without a break in the NICU for nineteen hours, handling
> one emergency after the next . . . with [a] neonatal attending who didn't
> seem to want to listen to reason. I was tired and frustrated and angry—
> angry at the nurse for ordering me around, angry at the hospital for not
> being air-conditioned, angry at the weather bureau, which I figured should
> be held responsible for the heat wave, angry at my medical school adviser
> for even suggesting that I look into the residency program of the Boston
> Medical Center . . . angry at this baby, who, in addition to everything else
> that was wrong with him, apparently didn't possess a single, solitary, visible
> vein within the confines of his entire body which would successfully hold
> a tiny butterfly needle. But most of all I was angry at myself for failing,
> angry because I couldn't get a simple IV started. (114)

Marion, like other writers, goes on to show himself eventually gaining the
skills and, usually, the equanimity that he lost that night. In the epilogue to
his memoir, however, he writes that

> the most psychologically damaging part of medical education in the United
> States today is, undoubtedly, the enforced life-style of our interns and
> residents. . . . This system is grossly unfair not only to interns and residents
> but also, and more important, to their patients, who should be cared for by

physicians whose senses and judgment have not been impaired by chronic, unrelenting exhaustion. (266–67)

Other writers also show themselves in moments of cruelty. William Nolen recounts the following incident:

I had been up most of the previous night and was operating on a short fuse. "Damn it," I shouted at her, "if you won't let me do this job you can bleed to death! I'm sick of your bellyaching." This, quite naturally, only made matters worse. Mrs. Ramos started to cry and became completely uncooperative.

Jean had been watching me from the nurses' station. Now she got up and walked over to the bed. "Dr. Nolen," she said, "there's some fresh coffee in the kitchen. Would you like a cup?"

"Thanks," I said, "I guess I will." . . . After a while I went back to Mrs. Ramos' bed, accompanied by Jean. It was obvious that she had spoken to Mrs. Ramos while I was in the kitchen. Jean held her hand while I did the cutdown and there was no rebellion of any kind. When I finished Mrs. Ramos said, "I'm sorry, doctor—I was just so scared."

"I'm sorry too," I said. "I shouldn't have lost my temper."

"I understand," Mrs. Ramos said. "Miss Swanson explained how hard you work." Jean made no comment. (73)

Nolen's apology to a patient is one of the few recorded in the memoirs. Even so, the role of the nurse, Jean, in calming Nolen while still defending him to Mrs. Ramos, plus Mrs. Ramos's own apology (notably, offered before Nolen's) are tacit acknowledgment of a physician's privilege, even in the face of grossly bad behavior.

Danielle Ofri seems to act without a nurse's objection when she orders an antibiotic to be administered in a purely punitive way: four syringes, every four hours, in the buttocks. Mr. Goode had repeatedly, and most rudely, refused to permit the insertion of a central line for administering his medications (a central line is a catheter placed through a vein to remain under the breastbone for quickly giving drugs): "I'd never actually hated a patient before, but Harold Goode managed to squirrel right in under my skin. Having crossed paths at that critical juncture in my training when I was first in charge, Mr. Goode was able to hone right in on my insecurities and make me feel incompetent" (129). Joseph Sacco offers neither apology nor excuse, but he also realizes (with the help, again, of a nurse) that he has gone over the line late one night in the emergency room:

> Suddenly, I became furious. An idiot kid who'd just started shooting up in total disregard to both himself and his family, who'd probably come within minutes of losing his life, and who was now slobbering all over his shirt, was telling the doctor he had done "nothing." I sat him up again and, holding him by the collar with one hand, slapped him hard across the face.
>
> "Wake up!" I yelled. "What did you take?"
>
> He didn't answer so I smacked him again, much harder, making him flinch. I was about to yell again when I realized that I was shaking. The nurse who'd been assisting with the patient looked up at me. Her eyes said she knew what I was feeling, and that she was feeling it too, but that it was time to stop. I released his collar, my hand still raised in the air, let him slump back down on the stretcher, and went to gather my things and go home, as my shift had ended. I never found out what happened to him after I left. (112–13)

The most heated depictions of anger expressed against patients appear in memoirs of the internship year, and often in the first half of that year, when young physicians are probably most uncomfortable with the responsibility they bear. Although such behaviors as those described above are never excusable—and the writers do not forgive themselves—it is important to note, especially with an eye to making medical education safer for both patients and students, that the most physically abusive treatment of patients by residents usually occurs when the resident feels the least confident and (even with an experienced nurse at his or her side) most alone.

The inhumanity of excessive work hours has often been criticized, both within and outside the medical profession. When a dramatic court case in New York in 1984 led the state to mandate maximum time requirements for residency programs, the medical profession itself stepped up its efforts to review workplace conditions for residents.[30] In the early 2000s the Accreditation Council for Graduate Medical Education (ACGME) established "common duty hour" requirements for the country's more than 8,300 residency programs. In summary, the requirements consist of an eighty-hour workweek, with one day off every seven days, no work day to extend longer than twenty-four hours (with an additional six hours permitted for didactic activities only), and ten hours of personal time after each work period, including call.[31] As residency programs come up for review and reaccreditation, they are cited if they have not met these requirements. In 2007 the ACGME reported, "The number of programs that are re-designing their patient care and education systems to adapt them to reduced resident hours continues to grow slowly."[32] Tensions around the new duty hours bring to a head the years-long tension between residents as workers in understaffed hospitals and residents as physicians still in an educational program.[33]

Less physically abusive to the patient but still psychologically harmful is a medical vernacular that casts patients as agents of punishment. Transue's earlier observation about *to code* (a shortening of the "code blue" often announced over hospital intercoms to alert staff to medical emergencies without alarming visitors) illustrates an attitude that pervades the casual language that students hear and come to use every day. Slang ranges from the cleverly depersonalizing to the cruel. Perri Klass offers the following gloss on med-speak:

> This special language contributes to a sense of closeness and professional spirit among people who are under a great deal of stress. As a medical student, I found it exciting to discover that I'd finally cracked the code, that I could understand what doctors said and wrote, and could use the same formulations myself. . . .
>
> And there is the jargon that you don't ever want to hear yourself using. You know that your training is changing you, but there are certain changes you think would be going a little too far.
>
> The resident was describing a man with devastating terminal pancreatic cancer. "Basically he's CTD," the resident concluded. I reminded myself that I had resolved not to be shy about asking when I didn't understand things. "CTD?" I asked timidly.
>
> The resident smirked at me. "Circling The Drain."
>
> The images are vivid and terrible. "What happened to Mrs. Melville?"
>
> "Oh, she boxed last night." To box is to die, of course.[34]

Steve Horowitz says, "I've heard doctors say, 'These people [drug addicts] are *not* human.' They call them SHPOZ, subhuman pieces of shit" (116). John MacNab defines *gomer* as "a nice old man" (191), but a few years later, in his first novel, *The House of God*, Samuel Shem defines the term as an acronym for the more hostile Get Out Of My Emergency Room, usually applied to patients who will only make life more difficult for a busy, tired resident (even if that patient might qualify as MacNab's "nice old man"—MacNab might have been well aware of the acronym, too, but refusing to give it credence)

(36). Scholars and medical educators write with some regularity about the uses of medical slang and humor, usually seeking to define the point at which humor turns from a benign coping mechanism to a dehumanizing attack.[35] Whether defense or attack, however, much of the dark humor heard among medical students and residents is a direct response to their own sense of powerlessness in the face of physical frailty and death.

Such an attitude is a tragic irony about power in medical education. It is a disquieting paradox that this damaging power is wielded by some of the people who feel most power*less*. Although some patients may distrust their physicians, most of them have no idea that *they* might be seen as a threat to a young clinician's fragile confidence or emotional stability, and they would be aghast to learn the power these neophyte caregivers attribute to them. It may be difficult for some medical educators to recognize (or allow themselves to remember) that the process of medical education could foster abusive behavior in its students or residents. It is easier to point to social or cultural bias. And the biases certainly exist, inasmuch as medical school is a microcosm of a society in which discrimination against less-advantaged people continues to flourish. To their credit, many medical schools include some curricula that address cultural biases in medical practice and in both undergraduate and graduate medical education. In addition, continued efforts to reduce the workload for residents addresses a major threat to the education of humane physicians. Given, however, the many facets of power differentials in medical education and practice, as well as an ongoing reluctance to talk head-on about power, most kinds of discrimination still exist. Moreover, however much shortened workweeks and reduced call schedules ease the *physical* exhaustion that is so debilitating to many students and residents, environments that continue to ignore the *emotional* strains faced by physicians in training—even when they are rested—will continue to be perceived as brutal by many. Educators who do not see the abuses of power felt by many of their own students may fail to generate an understanding of difference and power in all aspects of medical practice.

Relationships

OF ALL THE damages that power differentials can create in medical education and practice, the most troubling ones occur between medical students or residents and their patients. Although many pages of distressing relationships with patients fill these memoirs, there are also accounts of comfort, appreciation, and inspiration. These accounts suggest another story of medical practice, one in which physicians' work is grounded in and guided by countless relationships.[1] This story is often not recognized because the image of the solely accountable, self-sufficient, autonomous, and heroic physician still holds sway in the public imagination—and in the imagination of many physicians, even when their own daily experiences offer evidence to the contrary. Stories of nurturing relationships with patients, peers, and teachers run throughout most memoirs of medical education, and they offer a possible antidote to an educational process that is often described as alienating and hostile.

Throughout their medical education, students and young physicians are not only living in relationships with other people but are also explicitly thinking about those relationships in terms of their development as physicians. From the start, many students worry about how they will look to their peers, even when they question those peers' behavior. For example, Charles LeBaron and Michael Greger write, respectively, about the first and third years of their undergraduate medical education:

How long it took me to realize that when I was completely confused, chances were everyone else was too, that group silence meant group bewilderment, not comprehension. But Dumb Questions are rarely asked since no one wants to Look Foolish in Front of the Whole Class. (47)

It's not even about caring too much about grades, this self-deprecation. It's caring too much about what others think of you. Further, it's caring . . . about what people for whom you have no respect think of you. (22)

Later on, the self-reflection becomes more complex. Elizabeth Morgan writes about the effect that her fellow residents might be having on her attitude toward patients:

> I went to the kitchenette to pour out a cup of coffee, and sat down to think. The man had been stupid, provoking and rude, I told myself. All the same, I wasn't proud of the way I had behaved. It didn't seem right for me to speak like that, although all men surgical residents around me talked the same way whenever they were tired and irritated.
>
> I resolved to be a better doctor. I didn't like to think I was becoming unfeminine, but I knew I would not have spoken like that a year ago. (185)

In the past thirty years, the notion of relationships as a necessary and valuable aspect of human agency has gained prominence. In 1976 psychiatrist Jean Baker Miller developed a therapeutic method based on the premise that all human life is carried out within relationships, but that relationships, even intimate ones, are too often grounded within a society that gives unequal power to one of the members (usually men in couples). Miller advocated an approach to relationships that strives to identify and alleviate such differences. In 1982 Carol Gilligan published *In A Different Voice*, her now famous challenge to longstanding theories of moral development that held rights-based, independent-thinking judgment to be at the pinnacle of moral reasoning. Instead, Gilligan argued for recognition of an equally valid and sophisticated model of moral reasoning that was based on relationships and a sense of community.[2] These theories have had repercussions in the field of medical ethics, where the primacy of patient autonomy has been challenged by ethical models that emphasize community, negotiation, and context.[3]

Such arguments have led to a reconsideration of life writing as well. Well into the last half of the twentieth century, scholars of autobiography in the United States tended to treat the writing of autobiography as an exercise in establishing oneself as an individual, with an emphasis on seeing oneself as separate from others by virtue of achievements—and thus deserving to tell one's life story. With the advent of the civil rights and feminist movements, however, some historians and literary scholars began to challenge this seeming prescription for both writing and reading autobiographies. Among other things, they argued that autobiography was not the sole purview of the famous, thus opening the door for an appreciation of the life stories of "ordinary" people. They also argued that life writing was not necessarily an act of individuation, of seeing oneself as unique and separate in the world. They hailed writing, usually by women, which more often told the author's life in terms of relationships with other people, often a parent.4 Drawing on this work, autobiography scholar Paul John Eakin reexamined a number of autobiographies by famous men and concluded that their lives were also the product of their relationships with other people. In fact, he concluded, substantial parts of *all* autobiographies are about relationships.

To say that all people exist in relationship with other people seems to overstate the obvious. To make relationship the *starting* point in discussing the education of the physician, however, forces us to rethink the image of the physician as a medical Lone Ranger. Memoirs of medical education are all about negotiating relationships. One becomes a physician only by entering into new relationships on practically a daily basis. Memoirs of medical education lend credence to the theories of Eakin and other scholars, in literature as well as in moral development and psychology. In our broader society, not only have male/female, independence/relationship, and justice/caring long been cast as opposites, but the former qualities have usually been judged superior to the latter. Medicine has been caught on the proverbial horns of the dilemma created by these false dichotomies. The work of medicine may at times call for independent action and derring-do, but much of its work calls for deference, compromise, and teamwork. Blinded by the image of the heroic physician, however, medical education tends to emphasize singularity rather than community.

Peers

Nearly all aspects of learning in medicine are embedded in human relationships. The cadaver in gross anatomy, as I have already pointed out, has long been considered the medical student's first patient. Many students' imaginations create a personal relationship between themselves and their cadavers, but gross anatomy offers another important relational exercise: learning to work with other students. In some schools, medical students are assigned to a dissection table; in other schools, students select their own dissection partners. In either case, strong bonds are often formed among dissection partners, whether permanent or temporary, as reported by Dorothy Green-baum and Philip Reilly:

> Fern waved a quick good-bye and hurried across campus, trailing a scent of formaldehyde behind her. I knew I had not made a friend. "Well," I thought, as I shifted my anatomy book to my left hip, "we only work together. We don't have to like each other." (113) [Actually, the two women eventually become friends.]

> Over the months we had become close. . . . Now the four of us were meet-ing as anatomy partners for the last time. . . .
> Nancy had written a poem in honor of Kojak, which she wanted to read. I drew the black window shades. Paul flicked out all the lights, save for our overhead lamp. . . . We stood in the shadows as Nancy read. Then we quickly said good-bye. It was in the nature of medical education with its infinity of new rotations and heavy demands on one's time that the four of us never assembled again. (19–20)

These intense, often transitory, relationships in gross anatomy set the tone for much of medical education, particularly in the clinical years. In an earlier chapter I quoted Ron Maggiore's efforts to spend an evening in Chinatown with friends to celebrate the end of the third year.[5] Conversely, residency schedules can create an unlikely social circle, as Danielle Ofri notes about "liver rounds," a regular event for residents:

> I gazed at the motley housestaff swigging beers and laughing over chips and war stories. On the one hand, they were remarkably homogeneous—all high-achievers in their college and medical school classes, most middle class, white. The scheduling of residency, however, made people who would normally not ever socialize spend more time together than they would with even their spouses. (118)

Spending increasing amounts of time with people not of one's own choos-ing is not necessarily unique to medicine. Neither is irritation with com-petitive peers, but medicine has been almost stereotypical in its portrayal of cutthroat competition. Although complaints about the competitiveness of medical students have diminished in the memoirs over the decades, they have not entirely disappeared. When it is described, competition is never celebrated as a positive spur to one's own learning, but rather as a source of tension that can become destructive to everyone, as testified to by Ellen Lerner Rothman, Ron Maggiore, and Robert Marion:

> Alyssa sat in the center of the group, her eyes flaming and glassy with barely restrained tears. She held a sheet of paper and passed it around for the rest of us to see. The unsigned typed letter blamed Alyssa's competitive nature for damaging our class spirit and contributing to the atmosphere provoking our classmate's suicide attempt. . . .
>
> She could be aggressive in anatomy lab to do most of the dissecting, to identify the structures herself, to get her questions answered first. In this respect she was certainly not alone in our class, and perhaps people judged her more harshly because she was a woman. (35–36)

> There is a preponderance of gunner mentality: a lethal combination of pretentiousness and aggressiveness. This A type personality taken to the extreme creates a most hostile environment; animosity hangs in the air like storm clouds churning into some awful tempest.[6]

> I hated Phil Nirenstein. He was the kind of guy who always tried to outdo and outshine everyone else, to make himself look good to the discredit of others. He was easily the most competitive person I had ever met. . . . And ever since our first year of school, I'd wanted to kill the guy. (53–54)

Criticisms of competitive students are often linked to concerns that students who are less forward (although they may also be equally competitive) will be hampered in their own ability to learn, to do well, and to look good. The scramble to make a favorable impression on the infrequently seen attending physician does not always promote helpfulness and cooperation. The amount of time that authors spend talking about personal relationships with classmates, however, is relatively small, perhaps because friendship with one's agemates is the relationship with which they have the most experience. More anxiety-provoking to them is finding their way with patients and professors.

Patients

The relationships that loom largest for medical students are the ones with their patients. The least complicated of these, reported fondly by nearly all writers, occur when a patient acts as a kindly teacher. Philip Reilly describes the first time he was sent to draw blood from a patient's radial artery (in the wrist, just below the thumb), with a predictable lack of success:

> This time I apologized to Mr. Dobzhansky, took off my coat, rolled up my sleeves, and vowed one more try. Again, he assented. Again I felt the artery pumping at my finger. I plunged the needle firmly into this pulse and got back nothing. Defeat. Three sticks in a row had failed. What if this were an emergency? I felt totally incompetent.
>
> I could tell by looking into his eyes that Mr. Dobzhansky's wrist was hurting. Still, he did not complain. I was obviously more upset than he.
>
> "Sit down, son," he said. "Take a break. Get your nerve back. You can do it. It's just a bit tricky."
>
> Suddenly, it was like a boy with his grandfather. All pretense fell away. (122–23)

Often, a patient's helpfulness and support is a response to an earlier kindness. Robert Klitzman describes his relationship with Mr. Draper, which began when Klitzman chased down a dinner cart to swap Draper's meatloaf for the chicken he had ordered. "This small favor led him to view me as a friend," Klitzman writes, a favor that led Mr. Draper to make allowances later, when Klitzman struggles to measure the amount of oxygen in Mr. Draper's blood: "'Come on. Come on, doc. You can do it,' he rooted. My brow sweated. He was praying to himself, his lips twitching, urging me on. Finally, our eyes widened as a track of blood crept up the clear plastic tubing toward my tube. Discovering oil couldn't be a greater relief. The two of us grinned at each other; it was the only time he ever smiled in the hospital" (70–71).

Patients can buttress an unsure intern's confidence, as Ron Maggiore reports:

> Validation: the patient with metastatic breast cancer [bloggers on medschooldiary.com are careful not to use patients' names] was a sad case to behold. A 40-something-year-old woman with intraductal carcinoma with mets to her spine and knees with new onset of R hip/groin pain. New metastatic lesions on her R greater trochanter and iliac crest not present on hip films from 6 months ago. In our conversation about her disease and its insidious course, how she spends her day (the frenetic pace of the ER did not pick up at that time), she asked me about my goals. I said I am debating between rheumatology and oncology. In only 5 minutes into

our exchange, she looked at me and said very candidly, "You'd make an excellent oncologist." I was taken aback by this comment at first. I have had so much "constructive criticism" from attendings to make me a more efficient resident that we often do not seek the appraisal from our sincerest evaluators: namely, our own patients. I somehow mustered some sense of trust in those few minutes I got to talking to her.[7]

In these three instances, students and resident gladly accede power, which they were uncomfortable claiming at this point anyway, to someone who recognizes, sympathizes with, *and becomes protective of* the inexperienced physician.

Although many patients may be more forgiving of students' fumblings than students expect, most of them, understandably, have limits to their tolerance of awkward caregivers. Many patients may not be aware that students or residents are struggling to find a professional manner that is both respectful of patients and emotionally comfortable. Students and residents themselves are, usually, acutely aware of this and, while they understand why their patients are upset, they are often unsure how to redress the situation. Third-year student Ellen Lerner Rothman feels guilty when a patient to whom Rothman feels particularly close does not seem sufficiently happy or grateful after a successful surgery:

> I knew she was worried about her hip pain, and I understood that being in the hospital and nearly dying would not predispose most people to be on their best behavior. Nonetheless I was irritated with her. Why couldn't she acknowledge how sick she had been? Why couldn't she be thankful to be alive? I understood that her confidence in us might be shaken when we had medically certified her to leave, arranged for her to go, and then she suffered this life-threatening event. But I wanted her at least to be grateful that we managed to rescue her.
>
> But I also felt bad for feeling this way. How could I have all these expectations? What made me think that she wanted to share her experience of the day before with me? Why should I deserve that or consider it my right? (139)

Psychiatry resident David Viscott records the shame he felt when, in his frustration with a patient early in his residency, his offhand comments bring her to tears. Although his supervisor reassures him that he isn't a horrible psychiatrist or person, Viscott concludes,

I still felt miserable. I could hardly remember feeling lower. . . . I felt miles and years away from being a decent psychiatrist.

Also, my flip attitude was bothering me. I know I've already told you how it reflected my being unsure. But I didn't like to think that it got in my way to this extent. . . . What if Mrs. Sacks had taken my comment at face value and decided that no one could understand her? I would have done her a serious disservice. (62)

Sometimes in these instances patients become categorized as the punishing kinds of patients described in the preceding chapter, and the student or resident shifts blame for the testy relationship to the patient. John MacNab is aware of the danger of such a dynamic when he writes,

Another patient really made me feel stupid. Zella Rawson was 40 years old, black, the mother of three and in her fourth pregnancy. She had some third-trimester bleeding, and had been sent in for observation. She was up and around—too much so, because she was always at the nurses' station, with either a request or a complaint. The nurses disliked her and wanted us to send her home. She had been described in her chart as "manipulative"—I felt a kinship with the man who wrote that note two years ago. She complained about the tiny meals here and said she couldn't sleep because she was so hungry. She had my sympathy, and I wrote her an order for bread and butter to be given to her at night. Immediately after writing it I knew I had been manipulated. I don't know if it helped her sleep. In the course of her stay a very high blood sugar was noted. [They test Mrs. Rawson for diabetes, a process that causes her much discomfort. She is, however, eventually found to have diabetes mellitus.] As I wrote in the orders for the trial dosage of insulin, my orders for "bread and butter, h.s. p.r.n." mocked me. The next time a patient complains to me of hunger, I am going to sate him with 50 ml of glucose, and then administer the rest of the glucose tolerance test. Diabetes is one diagnosis I won't miss. Suspect everyone.

My mind moves to the right. (61–62)

In all three of these passages, the writers juggle their desires to like and be liked by their patients with their need to find a comfortable professional stance with these same people. They scrutinize the motives behind their behaviors, often turning that scrutiny upon their patients as well, and they begin to realize that becoming a physician often involves rethinking the rules of a trusting relationship, the nature of friendship, and the impossibility of a completely equal relationship with patients. As Emily Transue puts it, "The doctor-patient relationship is mutual but not symmetric. I can bring my emotions and personal life to it in limited ways, in ways that can help me to help her, but some fears are too raw for me to lay on the table. I can't risk putting her in the position of feeling she needs to help or comfort me" (113).

Troublesome in a different way are the sexual undertones that can occur in encounters between patients and physicians. Writers document a variety of such situations. Kenneth Klein describes his uneasiness with a patient, Gloria Milner, who seemed to be flirting with him:

> I asked her if she would unbutton her pajama top so I could examine her breasts and her heart. She unbuttoned the flannel shirt and threw it open. I checked her breasts and listened to her heart murmur. Then I tried to button her back together again. "Don't bother," she said.
>
> Next, when I asked her to pull her bottoms down just a bit so I could examine her belly she pulled them halfway to her knees. I tried to hike them up above her groin for decency, but she said, "What's wrong, Kenneth? You *are* going to be a doctor, aren't you?" I felt so stupid and helpless sitting on the bed with this woman whose pajamas were practically off. What if a nurse walked in? What if Dr. Hunter walked in? The situation was out of hand.
>
> I hurried through the rest of the exam. She finally buttoned her pajamas and then asked me to help her sit up. . . . "You know, Kenneth, you've been very kind to me. You have a very nice bedside manner. You'll make a fine doctor someday."
>
> I was confused about what was happening. I didn't like not having things under control. (167–68)

Ellen Lerner Rothman also links sexual or overly familiar gestures with the discomfort of not being in control of the interview, a response having as much to do with power as with sexuality. Rothman reports,

> My male patients often thought I, as a young, small woman, was cute. Some of the older men identified me with their granddaughters, and one patient even surprised me with a familial peck on the cheek as I left. But some of them used a distinctly more sexual tone. I preferred a slightly less formal tone in my patient relationships, but these attitudes made me uncomfortable. I never found a way to discourage this atmosphere from

creeping into my patient experiences. I even accepted it because these men were often willing patients and didn't complain about the two-hour histories and physicals I subjected them to. (72)

Rothman describes her decision to tolerate a clearly sexual tone in exchange for the access it gives her to patients' time, evidence that she feels more in control of her own feelings than Klein reports of himself at that time.

When the practitioner responds sexually to her or his patient, however, writers are nearly unanimous in their uneasiness. Melvin Konner describes one such instance in his third year of undergraduate medical education:

> The same day, the exquisitely beautiful teenager whom I had been unable to forget returned to the clinic, and this time she and her mother did end up in my examining room. She was still suffering from headaches. I could not remember ever being made so uncomfortable by a routine examination. She seemed already accustomed to the privileges and burdens of great beauty. Still, it would not do her any good to have a doctor who lost his marbles in her presence. Yet I was disoriented by her beauty, and even touching her seemed a violation of something sacred. Routinely putting my hand inside her blouse to get the stethoscope into place, so that I could listen to her heart and lungs—even with her mother looking benignly over my shoulder—seemed like the most outrageous act of sexual exploitation. (203)

Emily Transue writes at length about a relationship that developed over several months during her first year of residency:

> The thing I'm feeling now isn't a doctor-patient click. It's a different click. It's feeling that if I met this guy at a party, I would give him my phone number. . . . Nothing extreme, and yet it throws me completely, because I've never felt anything like this when talking to a patient before.
>
> A patient.
>
> You're not supposed to think these things about patients. . . .
>
> Let me be clear that I was not confused about how to act: ignore it and then forget it. The situation was not complicated. I just hadn't believed I could feel this way, and I do. (175)

The patient begins asking Transue personal questions, which she refuses to answer, only increasing his inquisitiveness. She refuses to tell him her age although she has told it to other patients who have asked, sensing a different tension here. The dynamic continues through subsequent clinic visits and occasional encounters in the hall. She concludes the chapter by saying that she has at least learned from this experience that sexual "chemistry" is still possible for her. She had been contemplating marriage to someone for whom her feelings were largely comradely because she had begun to fear that she lacked romantic passion, and now, at least, that fear has been allayed. Still, "someone who's not a patient, please, next time," she concludes wistfully (184).

Although most undergraduate medical education includes courses, usually preclinically, in what is called doctor-patient communication, clinical instruction on how to establish a personal relationship with patients seldom occurs. More often, students observe their teachers—and draw their own conclusions. The memoirs of undergraduate and graduate medical students contain many observations of physicians relating to patients in ways that the writers find appalling or admirable. On the negative side, examples from Michael Greger and Dan Imler:

> The gynecology-oncology attending stops outside the patient's room to tell the residents, "Let's make this quick." She tells the woman inside that she has a particularly bad form of invasive cancer and will need radical surgery and maybe chemo and radiation. The doctor continues to speak right through her sobs, talking about nodes and spinals. And then leaves while the patient is still crying. The secretary gives her some handouts on the way out. (74)

> Basically, the fellow [physician in postresidency training] asked opaque questions that didn't elicit any sort of patient perspective. All he got was that my patient was in a lot of pain (which is obvious if you [meet] him). Instead of talking to the patient about the source of his psychosocial problems, which are more detrimental to his daily life, the physician simply prescribed Zoloft (antidepressant) to improve his mood. Not once did he allow me to be involved in the process, even though I think I could have added a lot that he did not know. Very, very crappy![8]

Imler not only criticizes the fellow's behavior with the patient but also goes on to wonder if that could be himself one day: "Personally, I worry that maybe I'll fall into the same traps as this physician, more worried about my own life than theirs. There has to be a balance I guess, I hope I can find the right one." Ron Maggiore praises an attending physician in internal medicine who chastises a pathology resident, but also worries about his own fallibility: "One of the doctors had to ask the resident who was presenting to say the patient's name . . . I hope I don't completely forget that there are real human beings associated with these diseases and processes . . . [Maggiore's ellipses] not just a diagnosis or complication or a treatment cohort."[9]

On the positive side, Craig A. Miller describes an attending surgeon, Dr. Atcheson, who was operating when a resident inadvertently left a sponge in his patient's abdomen. Atcheson goes directly to the patient, Mrs. Gardner. After some preliminary conversation, he confesses:

> "I'm afraid I accidently left a sponge inside you. We saw it on the x-ray we took this afternoon. I can't explain how we missed it—this has never happened to me before. But we did. And we have to go back to the operating room and take it out. I'm sorry."
>
> There was a long silence as Mrs. Gardner's blue head absorbed the information. . . .
>
> "Well, you know best, doctor. I appreciate what you and your people have all done for me. I think you're trying to save my life."
>
> So that was that. Mrs. Gardner had decided that her doctor was doing his best and that human beings make mistakes. It was a great lesson for me, too, of course. Dr. Atcheson had treated the situation with straightforward, uncompromising honesty and—most importantly, I think—he had kept in close communication with the patient. (89)

In watching the attending physician on her intensive-care rotation during her undergraduate education, Audrey Young wonders how both family and physician are feeling:

> "That was the best thing," [Dr.] Cusack said softly. Later I realized he might be speaking not only for her but also for himself. I had seen him twice with patients who died so quickly that no one had time to say good-bye. I would watch him bring parents, spouses, children to face unexpected situations and usually under considerable time pressure. At first I could see only the artistry with which he handled such situations. Gradually I saw how affected he was by small failures between humans at the end of life, the tragedy of seeing people not speak in time. I could see now why we had tried from the beginning to predict the future, to prepare Milo and his family for this most difficult and protracted human process. (89)

When physicians in training see knowledge, skill, considerateness, and conversational ease all present in one physician, they usually conclude that the physician is also caring—or at least respectful—of his or her patients. What is deemed good communication between physician and patient does not necessarily signify authentic caring on either person's part. When it comes to observing physicians, however, watchful underlings seem to have a fairly accurate eye and ear for the genuine article. Significantly, however, authors rarely report conversations with these physicians about their emotions and relationships with patients. This silence about the personal dimension of medical practice is one of the biggest lacunae in medical education.

The personal, emotional dimension of the relationship between patient and physician is evident to most of the writers of these memoirs from their very earliest contact with patients. Some patients endear themselves to students and residents merely by resembling a family member. Mark Lee sees his own son and family in the following situation during his pediatrics rotation:

> I also met a little boy who was closer in condition to my son, Manning, than any other kid I have ever met. He had infantile spasms and intrac-table seizures his whole life. The same surgeon that did Manning's hemi-spherectomy had do[n]e a corpus colostomy on this boy and he had been seizure free for a few months until the week of admission. He was only a year younger than Manning and had many of the same characteristics. He was floppy and weak but had those big eyes that made him look like he was somewhere far away. Maybe a place that is better than here. His mom sat on the bed next to his crib and made him a balloon from a latex glove. She wrote "I love you" on it and I could feel the aching that I get in the back of my throat when I think about my kids and Manning especially. She had adopted him at birth. I felt like I knew what the years had been like for her and how probably most of her friends knew what sacrifices she made but they probably still didn't know what it was like for her at night as she lay in bed and listened to her little boy seize.[10]

Some writers find ties with patients they had least expected to identify with, as Emily Baldwin writes about her visit to a homeless clinic:

> In fact, I think that the most important things I shared with these men had little to do with medical knowledge or medical cures. What meant the most to me, and perhaps also to them, were the conversations we had about the commonalities that make us all human: the books that one man reads because he gets so bored during the day. The trick-or-treating one man did with his son. One man's descriptions of life in prison and what

could be done to reform the prison system. In the middle of the conversations, it mattered rather little that one of us was a medical student and one was a drug addict, and that recognition was the most powerful thing that I learned from that night.[11]

And sometimes the connection is one-sided. Frank Huyler describes performing a lifesaving emergency procedure so automatically that what he had done came to him "almost as an afterthought":

> Later that night, after my shift, I went to see him in the ICU. He was already off the ventilator and breathing on his own, waking up, coming back, making dim animal noises through a haze of morphine and Valium. I knew that he would leave whole, and I sat there in the dark for a while, watching the red and blue lights of the monitor, savoring him, taking something for myself. (57)

Nearly every author tells at least one extended story about a patient of whom she or he came to feel especially fond, even if that feeling wasn't reciprocated. For Steve Horowitz, one of those people was Anna Wilson. He introduces the relationship with the generalization, "Instead of battling for improvements, you end up fighting just to maintain the status quo. It can leave you cynical, almost always assuming the worst. . . . You don't want patients to die, but you certainly don't want them to die on your floor, on your service. You want to avoid all the hassle involved" (133–34). Horowitz's irritation, however, begins to lift the minute he enters his new patient's room:

> Anna Wilson was eighty-three, but didn't look a day over forty-five. She was black, about five feet tall and though she had obviously lost a lot of weight, somehow she still looked chubby. Cherubic, almost. Her hair was very fine, a little scraggly, and not a bit gray. It was dyed blacker than coal.
>
> But it was her eyes you noticed first. They were bright, glowing, alive. They moved all around, bouncing off the ceiling, the wall, the floor. Surrounding her eyes was a face that seemed ageless. She probably hadn't looked any different thirty years ago. . . .
>
> But underneath the voice, and the bubbling, and the warmth, Anna Wilson was frightened. Maybe you knew that because she kept putting off the questions. Or maybe it was because you knew the woman had cancer.
>
> Because she was afraid, I did not ask her questions that would make it obvious I was leading to cancer. Anna Wilson was too hip for me to be obvious. (134–35)

Horowitz's "you" in these opening paragraphs of his chapter suggests an impersonal distance between him and Anna Wilson, but he shifts to "I" as he begins to become fond of her. His examination of her and the various tests he orders over the next several days only raise the anxiety for both of them: "I was not going to give a label to her disease—at least not right now—or even tell her the possibilities. I wasn't going to take this lady's hope away from her. Damn it, I was going to *give* her hope if I possibly could. It was hard, though. She was too quick for her own good" (136).

When and how to tell the truth to patients, particularly about cancer and even more particularly when the physician realizes how much a patient may fear that diagnosis (or "label," as Horowitz says) is a perennial debate in medical ethics. Opinion these days falls more toward earlier disclosure, even of suspicions, than it did in the late 1960s and early 1970s of Horowitz's internship, but his desire to protect Anna Wilson and offer her hope seems to issue as much from Horowitz's growing fondness for her as from professional paternalism. Horowitz describes his growing personal involvement:

> While we were waiting for the [x-ray] results, I found myself making excuses to go into her room and talk to her.
>
> We didn't discuss medicine, or the tests. We talked about things we both enjoyed. She told me how she loved to be in the country when the leaves turned. . . .
>
> She talked about her fifty-five years as a city librarian and about her two daughters, one a schoolteacher and the other a doctor. She talked worriedly about her Vietnam veteran grandson who had become a drug addict. She talked about how her fourteen-year-old granddaughter wasn't doing very well in algebra. "Oh, my family, they *are* something," she'd say.
>
> And I opened up too, talking about things I had never discussed with a patient. . . .
>
> I shouldn't be talking about these things with one of my patients. But I couldn't help myself. I was captivated. . . .
>
> I wanted Anna Wilson to live, above and beyond being a doctor. It didn't have anything to do with not wanting to fill out forms or call the family. (136–37)

When the diagnosis of cancer is confirmed, Horowitz finds he cannot bear to tell Mrs. Wilson the bad news, but he couches his fear in hers: "I knew that the truth would break her," he writes, so "I was going to tell her in the most obscure terms possible. I was going to do it in the best traditions of medicine." Mrs. Wilson's unflagging faith in him as she finally agrees to the surgery she has so adamantly resisted only deepens his resolve to help her: "She brought my whole arm against her chest and smothered it inside of her, as if that was her only hope. I felt that way, too. I was her hope and I wasn't going to let her down" (138–39).

Horowitz takes a vacation day from his work to be with Mrs. Wilson the day of her surgery, and her continued faith in his support erases his doubts about being with her: "Inside, I started to cry. The hesitancy I had had about whether all of this was wrong, inappropriate for a doctor, dissolved. Schmuck, why would you even hesitate? You're a human being first, remember." Horowitz is there when Anna Wilson emerges from anesthesia, and in repeated visits he meets her family. He writes, "If I could make Anna that happy by having her know that a doctor—that I—cared, that was enough. Because at this point there was nothing else I could offer her." When she leaves the hospital for home, "It was a tearful goodbye, mainly for Mrs. Wilson. She thought she would never see me again. I bent down, kissed her and said to myself, I'll be seeing you again soon" (140–42). This time, Horowitz's shift from "Anna" to the more impersonal "Mrs. Wilson" represents his retreat to a more detached relationship.

When Anna Wilson eventually returns to the hospital, via the emergency room, she is dying:

> She didn't even look like Anna Wilson. She was much thinner than I remembered and her eyes looked sunken. She didn't have her teeth in and her hair was gray; the dye was gone. This woman's life had been drained out of her in six weeks.
>
> She was too immersed in her pain to recognize me, either. I bent down near her and, for the first time calling her by her first name, said, "Anna, Anna, this is Dr. Horowitz. You remember, Dr. Horowitz?"
>
> She was motionless for a moment. Finally I saw her eyes start to clear. "Dr. Horowitz," with a very low voice. "Dr. Horowitz, thank God I found you at the hospital again. I know you'll be able to help me."
>
> I put my hands over my face. I felt helpless. (142)

Although he is no longer working on the service to which she is assigned, Horowitz wants to be present when she dies, but he must go away one weekend and, when he returns, a different person is in Anna Wilson's hospital bed. Horowitz concludes this chapter of his memoir:

Why couldn't I at least have been there to say good-bye, to hold her hand? I felt cheated—of her friendship and of my right to help—and I felt angry. But most of all I felt empty. Drained. I wanted to cry or put my fist through a wall, but I couldn't summon up the emotions. I didn't have the time.

I returned to the ER, mechanically went about my job, saw the next patient, administered my medicine. I was already behind schedule. (143)

Horowitz the author has deliberately crafted this chapter to which he has given Anna Wilson's name. It opens with a statement about the cynicism of physicians called to take care of dying patients and concludes with intern Horowitz's hurried return to work, a busy schedule that, he believes, allows no time to think further about the death of Anna Wilson. Between those statements, however, Horowitz documents the emotional roller coaster he underwent in coming to care *about* his patient, as opposed to merely taking care *of* her. He doesn't ever say that it was wrong of him to have these feelings for Anna Wilson, but he repeatedly notes his inability to put these feelings into the context of his role as her physician. There is much food for broader discussion here about paternalism and its unavoidable presence in caring about a patient, and there will be differing opinions about Dr. Horowitz's attitudes and behaviors, even about his role in pressing for surgery that had little to offer Mrs. Wilson. For the purposes of this chapter, however, the important thing to notice is how the author shows himself repeatedly debating internally how or why he should feel or care about Mrs. Wilson. The gamut of emotions he feels upon finding her gone mixes professional and personal ego with a genuine sense of loss. Rather than taking the time to sort through these feelings, however, Dr. Horowitz allows the pressures of his overfilled schedule to give him an excuse not to think about them further at the time. Thus, author Steve Horowitz shows his readers the emotional cauldron in which all young physicians eventually find themselves and the ease with which their environment allows them to avoid grappling with these feelings.

Every memoir has at least one story about a patient like Anna Wilson. *Distance* is the term usually used in talking about how *close* a physician should be, emotionally, to a patient—a paradoxical term that already implies medicine's answer to that quandary. Memoirists repeatedly report being teased or criticized for, as it is usually put, caring too much for their patients. For example, from, respectively, Elizabeth Morgan, Robert Klitzman, and Kenneth Klein,

"By rejecting you she is externalizing her own self-rejection."

"Maybe," I said. "But it doesn't make it easier for me."

The neurosurgeon laughed. "Liz, you're a surgeon. You can't let these things bother you. You've got to be tough." (138)

Each day after visiting Judy, I ventured into the adjacent room, occupied by Mrs. Kunoshi Nakamoto, a slender Japanese woman with metastatic lung cancer. . . . For months she'd refused to see doctors, and drank a special herbal tea sent to her from relatives back in Japan. But the cough never left. "She's dying," Emmanuel had warned me on my first day. "Don't spend your time with the dead." (38)

On psychiatry it was finally OK to say you cared about patients without feeling like a softie. I loved it. (253)

Writers also report, although far less frequently, the physicians (residents or attendings) who support caring and shows of emotion. Two of the more striking examples were cited in the preceding chapter: the resident who comforted Emily Transue in her grief for a dying patient, and the resident who dropped his gruff tone when he encountered Robert Marion's tears over the dead child brought to the emergency room.[12]

More often, however, students and residents receive little support, even implicitly, for their emotional reactions to a patient's illness or death. Frank Vertosick Jr. uses the term "surgical psychopaths" to describe physicians whose "emotional numbness" toward their patients "progressed to the [point] . . . wherein one's humanity is placed under general anesthesia" (107). Several years into his neurosurgery residency, he found himself becoming "hardened . . . to death" and "cynical about suffering" (107)—or so he thought, until the death of Charles Bognar devastated him. Trying to repair an aneurysm (weakened segment of artery) in Bognar's brain, Vertosick's overly cautious approach caused the aneurysm to rupture, leaving the man with little brain function for the brief remainder of his life. When the surgery was discussed at the weekly conference for such cases, called "death and doughnuts" in his program, Vertosick was appalled that his angst was not shared by the more-senior residents and attending physicians: "The aneurysm ripped, the patient stroked out, tough luck." Although in part the lack of interest reflected their knowledge that Bognar would most certainly have died without the surgery, Vertosick was still upset that they did not respond to either the man's death or Vertosick's own grief: "I gazed about the room at the dozen or more staff surgeons present that morning, one hundred years of neurosurgical experience among them. Surely, these were ordinary men? Their learning curves must have devastated dozens upon dozens of lives. Why were they still sane?" (220–21). Vertosick was left to himself to decide against "surgical psychopath[ology]" (and to designate it as such [107]) and in favor of caring: "Caring makes the hands shake, but it also makes us dread disaster and work with every fiber of our being to avoid it" (225).

The creation of distance between oneself and one's patients is an often subtle process in hospital work. It can begin with the excitement of success-fully treating or diagnosing a patient's illness, as experienced by Danielle Ofri and Kenneth Klein:

> But as soon as I'd enjoyed my fleeting moment of pleasure—heightened, of course, by having done it in front of a group of awestruck medical students—the reality of the situation and the very reason why I was even putting in a central line flooded right back at me. After the bravado of slipping in the central line on the first try and suturing neat one-handed stitches, I was still left with an emaciated woman not much older than I who was about to die from something that I couldn't quite figure out, much less do anything about. (150)

> My excitement grew. I asked more questions and poked some more, trying to understand this malignancy. Was it a primary liver cancer or did it arise elsewhere and spread to the liver? I was hot on the trail of a tumor.
>
> Suddenly it occurs to me that this interesting diagnostic problem is a man with children and grandchildren and friends who love him. And it also occurs to me that this man will soon be dead. In my frantic effort to make a diagnosis, I forgot the meaning of that lump on the liver. I forgot that the tumor is not in a jar; it lives in Mr. McMaster's belly. He can't walk away from it at the end of the day as I can. To him it's not an interesting case at all—it's his death. (153)

Here, writers follow moments of personal triumph with the sobering real-ization of what that accomplishment means for the patient. Another frequently recorded opportunity to depersonalize patients is the substitution of a patient's name with a disease, organ, or room number, as Doctor X reports:

> With the kind of patient flow that we've been having . . . it is just amazingly easy to fall into the trap that always made me so mad in medical school

of regarding the patient, quite sincerely, as a leg, or a shoulder, or a gall bladder. . . . If any surgeon ever introduced *me* to a crowd of bright-eyed, wise-guy medical students as "this Stomach," I'd pick up the nearest blunt instrument and brain him with it. Yet I find myself thinking, and even recording in this journal, what we did with this Gall Bladder, and saying how Archie Everett had this Leg to fix. (292–93)

Every memoir contains at least two or three extended descriptions of students or residents using similar ways of depersonalizing their patients, sometimes in the forced rush of minimal contact and sometimes as a deliberate way to protect themselves from emotions that threaten to overwhelm them. Most of them, at least at the time of their writing, are aware—and critical—of this phenomenon.

The problem that faces most practitioners in establishing a workable emotional relationship with a patient—close enough to exchange fondness and concern but far enough to assess accurately a changing health situation—continues throughout the years of undergraduate and graduate medical education. Claire McCarthy describes how she came to realize how both therapeutic and personal relationships could—must, she argues—coexist:

The touching became easier, too. I worked at draining the personal from my fingertips, at concentrating on what I was looking and feeling for rather than on the patient. It was a matter of being there but not being there, of being present as physician, but not as peer or friend. That's not to say I wasn't friendly or that later I was never friends with my patients; it's just that doing physical exams requires some distance, especially at the beginning. (37–38)

The ability to move in and out of, for want of better terms, personal and professional feelings for a patient is probably the most accurate way to describe how many physicians come to negotiate the complex emotional dimensions of their relationships with patients. Physician and medical educator John L. Coulehan uses the phrases "tenderness and steadiness" and "emotional resilience" to describe a similar dynamic. Surgeon William Nolen describes the effort as a tightrope:

Heartbreak, sorrow, despair—they were part of our everyday life and we had to learn to live with them, to confront them, to be defeated by them—to bear them.

It was not easy. The obvious defense against the tragedies we encountered was to become indifferent, to do our job as well as possible and the results be damned. . . .

But it was equally important that we "care" for our patients in the true sense of the word. If we didn't become emotionally involved we wouldn't do our job as well as we should. We had to be, at one and the same time, compassionate and calloused. It was a difficult line to walk. (260)

How to enter into a positive emotional, caring relationship with patients is a central concern of nearly all the writers of memoirs of medical education. By far most of what they write details the joys and sorrows experienced in caring for patients. Here, *care* is emotional as well as technical. Although the writers vary in the degrees of closeness that are comfortable to them, they seldom seek complete emotional detachment from their patients. Usually, however, they struggle alone to find that position of comfort.

Professionals

Although relationships with patients consume most of the pages of memoirs of medical education, these relationships occur within the context of the writer's relationships with a bevy of health professionals. Central in the budding physician's mind, however, are the more-senior physicians she or he sees and works with. As writers describe their encounters with physicians, they inadvertently demonstrate the difference between a *role model* and a *mentor*. A role model is just that, a personage to watch and copy, without necessarily any personal interaction. Mentoring implies a more personal degree of interaction that is motivated by a desire to foster the successful development of one's charges. As students pass through the years of their education, they encounter more role models than mentors, due in large part to the fast pace and frequently changing personnel in clinical settings, but also because of the absence of mentoring as an explicit dimension of medical education. An article in the *Journal of General Internal Medicine* reports that 160 hours of observing hospital rounds of four ward teams showed attending physicians seldom responding directly to behaviors in students or residents that they later identified to the researchers as disrespectful of or hostile to patients. If they responded at all, it was in nonverbal gestures or comments that "avoided blaming learners."[13] (Contrast these behaviors with the descriptions of pimping, in which shame and blame are often implicit.)

In their earliest clinical rotations, students seldom report personal conversations with physicians other than jocular give-and-take in hospital hallways and conference rooms. From their years of undergraduate medical education, the writers' depictions are almost solely of the teaching dialogue, most of it intimidating and even demeaning, as reported in the previous chapter. In the later years of residency, closer relationships with faculty are more likely to be described, but still I found few that I would call personal friendships with attending physicians, even after the end of many years of residency. William Nolen writes about the physicians with whom he developed "close rapport" (178), but he also describes the special effort he made to situate himself in their good graces. "We all wanted to stay on the right side of the 'big three' and we worked hard to do so. We had to," he says. For Dr. Loudon, who rounded early in the morning, Nolen makes a point to have the charge nurse page him the minute Loudon arrives in the hospital, so that "just as he was stepping in to see his first patient, [Nolen would] materialize at his elbow" (168). Doctor X's musings reflect how he is beginning to feel his way with his supervisors: "Dr. Fuller has warmed up a little bit recently; he jokes with me now and we get along pretty well. And this morning Tuckerman opened up again, over coffee in the cafeteria, and started talking about his fishing experiences, and we had a good chat" (106).

It could be that closer relationships existed for these writers, but such a general lack of depictions of them suggests that they don't usually occur, especially considering that coming to feel a kinship with physicians is an important part of most writers' experience. It is a phenomenon that most of them find simultaneously reassuring and alienating. Such identification begins, quite innocently, with an uncertain student's need to belong. Elizabeth Morgan describes her happiness when she first feels "part of the crew on a small boat in rough water" (52). Stephen A. Hoffmann writes, "Everyone listened attentively, and even on my first day, I could see that there was a unique esprit de corps to the team. Because of the nature of the work—intense, unrelenting, and emotionally exhausting—the ICU team is more cohesive than any other team of interns and residents in the hospital. Sitting down behind closed doors helping to plot strategy for the patients under my care, I felt like a member of a secret, privileged sect" (68–69). Melvin Konner continues this image of physicians as a protective team:

I have been absorbed into the "teamness" of medical training. During my last few months on the wards I tried to be decent to the patients, but my bonds, my emotional energy—what the psychoanalysts call cathexes—were all with doctors and medical students and, to a lesser extent, nurses. Authentic human feelings flow among members of a team, and these create and stabilize the social organization. It is the job of this organization to deal with the patients, but the patients are outside of it. Relations with them should be smooth, cordial, and efficient, but they are certainly not personal. And increasingly as one's training goes on, one feels quite protected by the fact that their dependency, their frightening, unpredictable involvement with you, is dispersed among the team members. . . .

Disloyalty to the team is always dangerous, and it can be remarkably subtle. Too great an involvement with patients can in itself be sufficient to suggest it. This works not because you have "gone over to the enemy," to put it crudely—after all, patients are not the enemy—but rather through an implied accusation leveled against the other team members: I care more than you do for patients, therefore you do not care enough. Avoiding this implication helps to suppress at least some nurturing impulses toward patients. (365)

Doctor X identifies this sense of privileged fraternity as not only treacherous but also his motivation to write *Intern*:

Over and above the confidential nature of the doctor's relationship with his patient, there is an ancient unspoken code of secrecy surrounding the practice of medicine and the men who practice it. According to this code, what the layman does not know is all to the good; the work that doctors do, the way they do it, the kind of men they are and the way they become doctors must be carefully hidden from public knowledge. I am convinced that this attitude is wrong, and unworthy of the great profession that perpetuates it. (2)

One implication of such a "code of secrecy" is that all physicians, by virtue of their education, automatically become a part of that secrecy. The description of this closed circle often sounds like a circling of the wagons, a self-protective measure that resonates with the novice physicians' desperate need for control over the fast-paced events in their lives. This professional relationship, even at its most informal, is not one that encourages expressions of doubt, toleration of dissent, or motivation to change.

There are many excellent, dedicated physician-teachers in medical schools, and the roles they model are usually ethical and caring. Even the good ones, however, operate within a system that not only works against building helpful, mentoring relationships but also makes it easy to avoid broaching the more emotionally charged aspects of medical practice. The hierarchical structure of medicine and the busy schedules of attending physicians contribute to the lack of familiarity between attending physicians and the students and residents who look to them to learn, not only about diagnosis and medical reasoning, but also about the personal and emotional aspects of caring for patients. For those physicians who are unable to articulate how they have come to understand their work and the relationships that infuse it, in fact, the environment in which medical education occurs *allows* them to teach form but not substance to students who crave the latter as much as the former.

Although physicians are central to the imaginations of students and residents as they look to their own professional evolution, much of the work of medical education takes place alongside other health professionals. The hospitals and clinics where physicians train are, foremost, working environments, where medical education is often disruptive and inefficient. Medical students and residents, the latter at least until they have been around long enough to fit into the daily routines, are welcomed with varying degrees of tolerance by the paid professionals who are not directly responsible for their education.

Nurses in particular hold a special relationship to physicians in training. Most nurses have greater medical knowledge than do medical students and many junior residents. They also usually have a greater knowledge of the patients on a service because of the more regular and intimate activities of nursing care. Memoirists write often, and often colorfully, about their relationships with nurses. There are those students or residents who see nurses as adversaries, as Craig A. Miller does in this instance—

The nurse found me in the middle of the procedure and basically treated me the way I would have expected to have been treated in adolescence by my mother if she had found me with a cache of porno magazines. What was I thinking? If there was a problem, why didn't she know about it? Why wasn't she "in the loop"? She tried to make me feel guilty for having performed a necessary procedure in her absence! My answer was perhaps unnecessarily combative, I admit; something along the lines of, "Sorry, I'm new here; I didn't see you on the unit and I don't know where the coffee break room is . . ." [Miller's ellipsis] (146)

—and those who see them as allies, as does Melvin Konner—

By the middle of the next week I was becoming comfortable with the process of labor and delivery, had made friends with all the nurses and most of the doctors, and was more help than hindrance in the labor and delivery rooms. The nurses on the floor seemed pleasantly surprised at a medical student who was not arrogant, who was interested in normal labor, who was willing to spend time with laboring women, and who—strangest of all—was plainly respectful of nurses. (215)

The wisest students and residents seek nurses as teachers, as did Stephen A. Hoffmann: "I recognized in Ellen a great teacher. It didn't take long for me to realize that I could depend upon and trust her judgment, and soon I invited her opinion right out" (226–27). Gender can both help and hinder the relationship between student doctor and nurse. Some female nurses are reported to favor male students and physicians, but the reverse is also recorded in these memoirs. There are undoubtedly times when clashes of personality and attitude are interpreted as gender problems. Finally, despite the stereotype of female nurses as willing sexual partners for licentious male medical students and residents, nurses as sexual objects figure in only a small number of the memoirs.

Students and residents portray their relationships with nurses more often than they do those with other health professionals. Formally designated *healthcare teams*—interprofessional groups created deliberately to work in a model of nonhierarchical professional cooperation—occur most often in gerontology, rehabilitation medicine, and hospice care. These kinds of teams are seldom portrayed in memoirs of medical education. All hospital- and clinic-based patient care, however, depends on the coordination and contribution of numerous health professionals. Medical education, although it usually gives at least lip service to this broader concept of teamwork, still organizes its clinical education along strongly hierarchical medical lines, a model that in practice does not permit much egalitarianism. The image of a gaggle of medical students and residents following the swift-stepping attending down the hall further reinforces the singularity of medical authority in many young physicians' minds, however limited or anachronistic it may be.

Family, Friends, and Fun

The comfort and hazards of medical "teamness" also have ominous repercussions for the private lives of physicians. I have already documented the effects of the pressured, demanding work of medical education on students' and residents' relationships with family members, partners, and friends. Writers have described how their social worlds come to draw more and more exclusively on the company of other students and physicians. Here, I shall add only a few passages from the memoirs that show writers thinking specifically about the effect of their educational environment on social and personal relationships.

The most frequent reports of social gatherings of medical students and, sometimes, their friends and family, come from the first two years of undergraduate medical education, when students are usually all in the same location and have easy contact with each other. Brian Hartman, Ron Maggiore, and Perri Klass, respectively, provide three such examples:

> Tonight we hit the fourth floor of Circle Center Mall in downtown Indianapolis. The place is called World Mardigras and it's a combination of four bars. We got in free and didn't have to wait in line by flashing our medschool IDs. Talk about a cool experience. It was fun seeing everyone out and having a good time while relieving all the stress of school. These are the people you go to class with every day and learn the science behind doctoring. You discuss possible treatments for patients we come across and debate ethical issues. It's awesome to see that everyone can then come together to celebrate the end of the first semester.[14]

> Last Wed., in much anticipation, I went with a group of classmates to see "The Vagina Monologues" being performed in Lincoln Park. . . .
>
> It was a fun time, a more edifying jaunt than the constant let's-get-smashed-again types of get-togethers our class board sloppily throws together to try to get students to know one another more . . . [Maggiore's ellipses] sadly, it's become hackneyed and I think many students are looking for better things to do th[a]n sit and get shit-faced with some random Joe from class.[15]

There is a married students' association at the medical school, but they are not eager to have students who are only engaged (much less just living together) come to their functions [Klass is clearly writing from an earlier time]. So one day a medical student gets up in front of the class and announces the first Living-in-Sin Potluck.

(In medical school, the potlucks are nonstop. Off-campus potluck, women's potluck, housewarming potluck—no one should go to medical school without a couple of really reliable recipes.) And so "those of us who are sharing these special years with someone to whom we are less formally bound," as the organizer says, honor our partners and each other one evening in the spring. And the medical students complain about medical school, and the partners complain about living with medical students, and a good time is had by all.[16]

Whitenton describes one of the rare social occasions for both family and peers, but it is a significant mark of her growing identification with medicine that her family leaves but she stays on. Writers are often aware that maintaining close family relationships becomes more difficult for them, from pressures both they and their peers generate. Ron Maggiore, whose family lives in a far Chicago suburb, complains, "That evening, yeah, like 9:30 or so, my roommate dropped me off at Union Station . . . I promised my family I'd be home this past weekend . . . [Maggiore's ellipses] having a 12-year-old brother is unique and some classmates just don't understand that you have to spend some time with younger siblings and not let them believe that you're alienating them by not being at home EVER."[17] Jamie Taweel feels guilty when he realizes he doesn't want his family to visit:

> It's the worst feeling in the world to be behind in your studies. It all comes so fast to you, that if you slip up one day, you pay for it in the end BIG TIME. . . . But my body is telling me that if I pull another late night, I'm seriously going to pay for it this weekend.
>
> The only problem is that this weekend, when I'm supposed to be catching up, my parents and brother are coming to town for the white coat ceremony. I feel so bad because I really don't want them to come out here. That sounds bad—let me rephrase it. I really want them to come out more than anything. But the fact that I have to entertain them is going to cut into my study time considerably (even if I leave them for a while and go to the library.)[18]

And Emily Baldwin struggles to explain (to herself as much as to her readers) how she negotiates the various relationships in her new life:

Today after lab a few of us went out for drinks at a bar near school. It was fun to hang out with people outside of class, which I haven't really done much, but as a result it also made me realize that I have been kind of antisocial since starting medical school. It's not intentional on my part, really, but I did start to think about my reasons. . . .

I know that if I'd just moved out to San Francisco by myself, after graduating from college, I'd be a lot more focused on making friends in my class. Instead, I find myself pretty focused on how to sustain the relationship I've been in for five years, and how to maintain some kind of circle of friends outside of school. I don't know if this is better or worse than turning to my classmates for close friendship, but it definitely is different. Most of all, I just worry sometimes that my classmates might think I'm being intentionally aloof, or that I'm missing out on opportunities to get to know these people who I probably would really like.[19]

The flip side of Baldwin's coin falls to students who are trying to figure out how they can ever find a partner, given the demands on their time and the increasing narrowness of their social circle. Brain Hartman's diary is a saga of finding and losing girlfriends, but his determination to find a permanent relationship never flags even as his frustration grows. He describes the dilemma thus:

Dating. That's the topic by request today. I could just say it's extremely hard and rare and just move on, but I don't think that would satisfy the curiosity.

When I got the acceptance to medical school, I had been dating my girlfriend for about a year and a half. Things were great and I was wondering about the whole long-distance thing since she was probably not going to be in Indiana. Then we broke up at graduation and I entered medical school single. I figured that is the ultimate pick-up line to use. Now that I've been here a year I know it's actually a pretty bad one.

The vast majority of people you meet during the year are in your class. I only go out with friends on the town about once every three weeks, and then we're all partying as a group, not trying to meet people. A lot of hookups happen through friends of friends, but most of us aren't in contact with our non-medical friends very often so that route is pretty much shot.

What it all boils down to is that it's very hard to start dating in medical school. The people in my class are mostly either married or dating someone and besides that you see them every day all day long, not really something you want in a relationship! The best route I've seen is, pathetically, at the library. There's a good intermingling of students there (medical, nursing, law, physical therapy, dental) who are all in the same boat. . . .

Now when people ask me what I do, I say I'm in school. If they persist I say I'm in medical school. I don't want to meet people who are attracted to the medical professional thing. Besides, if people were thinking clearly they'd realize doctors in general are not a group of people you should rush out to marry because of the time issues involved. Actually, I should mention that when I was on the cruise I told everyone I was in medical school, but that's a different story :)[20]

Not having an intimate relationship to allay the stresses of medical school, even with the acknowledgment that these relationships are often unfair for the partner, can be an isolating, alienating experience for people who don't want to be alone.

Incorporating new friends into one's life, particularly upon entering a new educational or work setting, is, again, nothing unique to medical students. Watching them think about the nature and priority of these relationships, however, underscores the centrality of relationships to these people's private and professional lives and the impossibility of drawing a line between the two realms. A medical education that is blind to or uncomfortable talking about the power of human ties in a physician's work misses the opportunity not only to address one of its students' greatest concerns but also to build on some of the strongest motivations that draw young men and women to the practice of medicine.

Conclusion

THE FOLLOWING POSTING from Dan Imler's blog, about five months into his third year of medical school, echoes many of the themes of the preceding chapters. Imler writes about his emotional struggle with the death of a young man a few days earlier. He reflects upon degrees of involvement with patients, his frustration with physicians who "don't care" and his respect for those who do, and his realization that he shouldn't ignore his emotions. He writes,

> It's been a tough week for me here in the PICU [pediatric intensive care unit]. . . . On[e] of the patients that I have been taking care of for the last week died yesterday. It of course is terrible when anyone dies, even more so when it is a child, but what made this one so bad was that it was so sudden and unexpected. I wrote about this patient in my last diary, he presented with liver-kidney-heart failure all presumably from his lupus, which was thought to be mild, and under control. He was 17 years old.
>
> I know that it might seem selfish to write about my own feelings when it is the poor child who has lost so much, but I think that for this venue having others understand part of my experience is probably the best plan. . . .
>
> I had gotten to know this child; I had become friends with the family. I knew what kind of music he like[d] and what he wanted to be when he grew up. It's amazing how much patients can become a part of your lives.
>
> Through medical school there seems to be an unwritten rule that you are to care about your patients BUT NOT TOO MUCH! What I mean is that you shouldn't become so close to them that you lose your objective bystander status. Then suddenly you are plopped into the middle of REAL LIFE and here you are taking care of someone who is becoming your friend like it or not. So I say sure it is important not to let yourself

become so emotionally involved that it affects your judgment, but I say that you should be much more wary of the opposite happening. I'm sure everyone has their horror story about some physician who just didn't care and left a patient behind.

Residents who care are great! And I was lucky to be around some who truly did care. They knew this was my patient and they were there to share how each of them had their own patient who was going to stick with them the rest of their lives. Just to expand on that, it is so true that certain patients somehow become "yours." No matter who else takes care of them, they are still yours and everyone knows it. It's so special and so scary. You become their steward and when something bad happens to them, it's as if something bad happens to you.

Ever since my patient died I haven't felt just right. Something has been missing! I think tonight though I was able to figure out what it was: Perspective! Soun[ds] silly, right, but here is what I mean. In the moment you are so caught up in whatever tragedy or triumph that you cannot see what is happening or what it means. For me, the devastation of death ruled me in an emotional confusion until I could grasp the meaning to me of what this horrible event meant. I needed to know that life is not governed by laws AND/BUT is not completely random. Things occur that I have no control over, but as long as I act true to my own self I can know that the world around me is chaos at MY discretion.

Enough reflection for now, we all know that I cannot begin to express the feelings of this event although I feel as if I have tried. My only advice for those who have yet to experience the death or sickness of YOUR patient is: Just don't hide from your own feelings. I know that sounds too touchy-feely, but honestly this is the time in your life when you need that. The worst thing I can imagine is myself refusing to deal with what I feel. When that happens you're just surviving life, not experiencing it. Can there be anything worse in this world?

Yea, time to call the therapist Danny-boy. Upp, here's that number on my speed dial, now how come it made it there . . . [Imler's ellipsis] [1]

Imler demonstrates here what I have come to call *emotional honesty*. In medical education it takes two forms: directed inward, it entails admitting one's feelings and thinking about their implications; directed outward, it entails expressing one's feelings and acknowledging those of other people. The former fosters self-reflection; the latter fosters a pedagogical method that attends to the emotional as well as the technical and intellectual development of physicians.[2]

Exercising both forms of emotional honesty ought to be easy. In an environment that disparages anything that might be perceived as weakness, however, emotional honesty may be one of the most difficult things to achieve. Conversations, let alone courses, that turn to talk of emotions are often dismissed as "touchy-feely," even when students feel a need for them from time to time, as did Imler in the face of his patient's death. After reading and rereading these memoirs of medical education, I would say that, although individual authors deal variously with power, relationships, and the embodied nature of medical education and practice, all of them suffer at one time or another from a debilitating sense of emotional isolation that could have been recognized, respected, and addressed.

Sometimes this kind of teaching does occur, as evidenced by Imler's "Residents who care are great!" But such teaching is usually informal and serendipitous. Moreover, I would be the first person to admit that a course titled Emotional Honesty would be a disaster. Imler, however, uses language, probably unwittingly, that suggests two ways in which emotional honesty could be integrated into medical education. First, when he states, at the end of his posting, "Enough reflection for now," he ventures into an area with which medical educators are more familiar, as *personal reflection* becomes almost a buzzword in many of the courses I shall describe in this chapter. Second, he unwittingly links emotional honesty to narrative voice when, at the end of his entry, he shifts to a self-mocking tone that allows him to retreat from his uncharacteristically confessional mode. For the remainder of this book, I shall consider the interplay of reflection and storytelling as one possible means for bringing emotional honesty into medical education.

Magical Thinking in Medical Education

Throughout these chapters I have deliberately avoided using the term *empathy* because of the wealth—more like a glut—of discussion that surrounds the term. As a keyword in the search engine PubMed, *empathy* generates 8,961 articles and books published from 1950 through February 2007. Counting only English-language articles about medicine (nursing and all other health professions are included in PubMed), over fifty references appear for the four months September through December 2005. I do not intend to recount or assess this vast scholarly discussion, other than to note that empathy certainly plays a role in what I have talked about in the preceding chapters as compassion, care, emotional honesty, connectedness.

For my purposes, I offer only one of the many definitions of empathy, by Howard Spiro from his widely cited article "What Is Empathy and Can It Be Taught?" Spiro describes empathy as an "almost magical phenomenon," a "feeling that persons or objects arouse in us as projections of our feelings and thoughts."[3] Spiro's choice of the phrase "almost magical" may have been canny or prescient—or both. Isolating the human impulses or gestures by which empathy "works" and devising ways to successfully instill them in physicians continue to elude medical educators—and not surprisingly, given the diverse backgrounds of today's medical students and the variety of ways in which they experience and express emotions. Sometimes the goals of these courses seem so self-evident as to be deemed unnecessary. In her memoir about coming to an understanding of death through her work as a transplant surgeon, Pauline W. Chen reports her and her classmates' response to the physician who concluded a lecture on communication with the statement, "You'll be a better doctor . . . if you can stand in your patients' shoes." Chen relates, "The entire class fell silent . . . because we believed that her statement went without saying. Most of us viewed ourselves as different from the old guard, *her* generation of physicians, those wise but hopelessly old fuddy-duddies" (167). The point of Chen's essay is that for her what might have gone "without saying" became much more difficult when the time actually came.

This passage, however, emphasizes that teaching about the emotional dimensions of medical practice often falls on deaf ears, even among would-be supporters. At other times, complex notions are reduced to such a common denominator that they become objects of ridicule, as they are in one of Vincent Lam's award-winning short stories, when a resident interviews a patient handcuffed to a stretcher in the emergency room:

"I am Dr. Fitzgerald," I repeated. In medicine we pretend that our names may be enough to control a situation.

"Breathe," I said. I sat on the edge of the stretcher, next to Eli's cuffed ankle. *Always sit down with the patient,* I was taught. *It makes it seem like you've spent more time and that you care.* In a chair, on the stretcher. *If you give this impression* (this is the subtext) *then the patients will do what you say and leave quickly.* I liked the stretcher, since sitting on the edge of the bed is what everyone's parents once did. *Where is it sore, dear?* "Speak–slowly. How–did–you–cut–your–head?" *Speaking slowly and loudly transcends both agitation and language barriers.* Another clinical pearl. (168).

In addition to the difficulty of teaching courses about interpersonal communication and relationships in a curriculum that places its highest priorities on "hard facts" and technical skills, educators of more humanistically focused material struggle to design courses with intellectual integrity for students who range widely in emotional sensibility and openness.

Whatever the seeming preference for facts and skills, however, since the late 1960s medical schools have regularly expressed a desire to instill or sustain humanistic values or behaviors in their curricula. In 1984 the Association of American Medical Colleges (AAMC), one of the accrediting agencies for undergraduate medical schools, included in its recommendations for the General Professional Education of the Physician (GPEP) that schools design educational programs that will foster the development of "desirable personal qualities, values, and attitudes of physicians." Included among these qualities are "stamina, moral sensitivity and integrity, curiosity and creativity, the ability to cope with intellectual and emotional demands, and a commitment to help and work with others." It recommends changes in the process of medical school admissions; calls for "faculty members [to] exhibit the personal qualities, values, and attitudes that they desire for their students"; and recommends that the workload of residents be "reassessed in light of the detrimental effects that [it] may have on the students whom they teach" and that, consequently, attending physicians spend more time with students.[4]

The AAMC became even more specific fifteen years later, when another group was assigned to elucidate the qualities they wanted graduating physicians to possess. The resulting Medical School Objectives Project (MSOP) calls for graduating physicians to be altruistic (listed first), knowledgeable, skillful, and dutiful. The first of these includes a number of behaviors related to nondiscrimination, advocacy, and justice. In their broad definition of altruism, MSOP includes "compassionate and empathetic in caring for patients . . . trustworthy and truthful in all of their professional dealings . . . integrity, honesty, respect for patients' privacy, and respect for the dignity of patients as persons."[5] That same year, the Accreditation Council of Graduate Medical Education (ACGME, the AAMC equivalent for residency programs) released its own document, the Outcome Project, which outlined the minimum program requirements for accreditation of a residency program. The six desired outcomes, usually referred to as *general competencies*, begin with "patient care that is compassionate, appropriate, and effective for the treatment of health problems and the promotion of health." Other competencies for residents include "interpersonal and communication skills that result in the effective exchange of information and collaboration with patients, their families, and health professionals," and "a commitment to carrying out professional responsibilities" such as "adherence to ethical principles . . . compassion, integrity, and respect for others; . . . accountability to patients, society and the profession; . . . and sensitivity and responsiveness to a diverse patient population."[6]

Although these accrediting bodies call for such humanistic attitudes as compassion and altruism, they do not specify how these goals (or the goals of any of the competencies) are to be achieved. The medical literature contains a wealth of reports on courses and programs that would address these goals. The following is a small, informal sample of these offerings:

The Patient Navigator Project, which sent first-year students into a cancer clinic to accompany patients and observe their interactions with physicians;[7]

Reflection Groups, in which third-year medical students in an ambulatory care course kept a journal that included "their personal reactions to their . . . experiences" and met regularly "to reflect on the emotional challenges of learning to be a doctor, in general, and of developing relationships with patients, in particular"[8];

Creative Projects, in which third-year students in an internal medicine clerkship created an original work of writing, art, music, or mixed media as a means to "reflect upon some encounter with a patient or other personal experience during the clerkship . . . that had made a significant impression, positive or negative"[9]; and

Art, Chaos, Ethics, and Science, a regular, voluntary dinner-discussion for faculty, residents, students, and nurses in the emergency department in which participants respond to a wide range of readings (including fiction, poetry, and memoir) in discussions of issues "typically outside the scope of the regular academic curriculum" and "to encourage reflection on our roles as caregivers on a personal, public health, and political level."[10]

In the description of all of these activities, the term *reflection* appears repeatedly, and most of them rely upon oral or written stories. All the authors reported success with their programs, although not all of them continued to be offered. Creators of the Patient Navigator Project, for example, reported that scheduling problems prevented the implementation of the project in subsequent years. Some courses are closely tied to the interests of one or two instructors, which could be a problem for the continuation of a course. On the other hand, such tenuousness underscores the individual nature of teachers as well as students and suggests the value of encouraging faculty to teach from their strengths and particular interests.

Some of the course creators argue that their programs serve not only to sustain or foster compassion or empathy for patients but also to alleviate the emotional isolation felt by many medical students and residents. The memoirs that I have cited here repeatedly link students' and residents' ability to feel and express compassion toward their patients with their own emotional stability at any one time. Whatever the value of humanistic courses, an environment that distresses its students will work against the goals of GPEP, MSOP, or the Outcome Project. In 2005, *Mayo Clinic Proceedings* published a review of over one hundred articles about stress in medical education, which has long been closely tied to the rise of cynicism, loss of idealism, and loss of empathy over the four years of undergraduate medical education. In addition to recommendations for better identification of students who are having academic and emotional problems, the authors recommend creating a "nurturing learning environment" for students. To do so, however, may also require the creation of a similar environment for residents and faculty who exhibit such behaviors as "disrespect, hostility, and rudeness." Two other recommendations are "promotion of self-awareness" by, among other things, using peer discussion groups "for students to express, analyze, and share feelings, which . . . helps students realize that their struggles are not unique"; and helping students "promote personal health," which includes getting "adequate sleep," seeing a physician regularly for both physical and mental health, and presentations that address how to maintain a "work-life balance."[11]

In short, curricular reforms have not eliminated—may not even have greatly reduced—the negative effects of stress in medical education, a finding that is borne out throughout the years of the memoirs of medical education I have examined. Moreover, the authors' appeal in the article in the *Mayo Clinic Proceedings* for nurture in the face of competition or disrespectful teaching behaviors, for self-awareness about and discussion of emotions, and for the promotion of the students' own health echoes the pleas of the memoir authors for the past forty years. Although many of the courses and activities now available in medical education were created to foster more-healthful environments, they still have a long way to go, for reasons over which their creators may have little control.

Emotional Honesty in Medical Education

Although the courses summarized above often used first-person oral or written storytelling, this was not their primary focus. Consistently, though, the courses' creators note the value of sharing personal accounts of emotional experiences as a means for better self-understanding and for lessening a student's sense of shame and isolation for possessing these feelings. Courses designed specifically to use stories—either the reading or the writing of them—to these ends report similar results. Three courses that more directly address the role of written narrative are described below.[12]

REFLECTIONS ON GROSS ANATOMY   This course began as a selective (one among a variety of short courses from which students are required to select) for first-year students within a larger course—Patient, Physician, and Society—at Northwestern Medical School. Its creator, physician Douglas R. Reifler, designed the course because he believed that most medical students dealt with their emotional responses to dissection "without much time or attention," resulting in unhelpful ways of dealing with the "human dimensions" of gross anatomy (184). He designed Reflections on Gross Anatomy to give students an opportunity "to explore and express their personal reactions to gross anatomy and to exercise their capacity for empathy by composing fictional accounts from their cadavers' perspectives" (184). Reifler used literary works relevant to gross anatomy by writers such as William Shakespeare, Ernest Hemingway, and Richard Selzer to generate discussions about death, bodily decay, and the contexts of the lives of people who have died.

Reifler gave students writing assignments during the second, fourth, and sixth weeks of the six-week course. Students were given two options for each assignment, some of which were as follows: "Describe on sensory, cognitive, and emotional levels the first incision into your cadaver"; "Describe, in your cadaver's words, the experience of dissection"; and "Write an autobiographical sketch of your cadaver's life (in the cadaver's words). Base your details on physical evidence" (187). Reifler carefully designed the assignments to shift the writing from the students' to the cadavers' perspectives, to bring them into an imagined relationship with their cadavers, and to encourage a direct consideration of death and dying. Students read and discussed their stories with the other students in the selective.

Reifler reports that the course succeeded in addressing some of the emotional components of gross anatomy, but he also credits the writing with giving students a broader language for thinking and talking about medicine:

> Most of these stories are clearly fictional, and the students understand that they do not accurately reflect what actually happened to their cadavers. Nevertheless, the students have developed their abilities to work with narrative accounts of human experience. The seminar has fostered an awareness of ways to describe human lives alternative to the usual language of medical records and oral case presentations. (195–96)

Although Reifler acknowledged that the special characteristics of his small group of self-selected students may have affected the success of the course, curriculum directors were sufficiently impressed with his results that two of these writing assignments were made a part of the curriculum for all first-year students.

THE PARALLEL CHART   Physician Rita Charon has been having students write narratives about patients for over twenty years, one part of a larger vision of medical education and practice that she has come to call *narrative medicine*. Charon draws her vocabulary from literary studies, in which she holds a PhD and in which she finds narrative elements and interpretive skills that directly parallel the human contexts of medical care. Time and plot, for example, can be discovered in medicine's concern for, respectively, the onset/duration of illness and causality. Identification with characters in a novel can help one think about intersubjectivity and ethics in relationships with one's patients.[13] Such exercises culminate for Charon in the "parallel chart," a private record in which students write about the kinds of things that are important to them but that they are not allowed to write in the medical chart, such as, "if your patient dying of prostate cancer reminds you of your grandfather, who died of that disease last summer, and each time you go into the patient's room, you weep for your grandfather" (156).

Charon asks her third-year students at Columbia University College of Physicians and Surgeons to keep a parallel chart during their clerkship in internal medicine. In her role as preceptor, Charon meets with her students (as do other preceptors) for ninety minutes, three times a week, for five weeks. Once a week, however, unlike the meetings led by other preceptors, students read from their parallel charts, and Charon responds to both the literary and emotional aspects of their stories. The two components are closely related, obviously, as "in the course of writing about patients, of course, students write a great deal about themselves. The patient's biography is always braided with the student's autobiography" (157). Charon is careful, however, to differentiate between what she does with her students and a therapy session, and she emphasizes the rigor of learning and applying narrative skills to medical discourse. She describes how the students' writing process takes them through an exercise of constant shifting between imaginatively revisiting a story and consciously working to convey that engagement to readers, a process that often brings the writer to a fuller understanding of those events and their impact on the writer. In addition, Charon has discovered that both writing in and discussing their parallel charts was often experienced as a "safe harbor" for her students (172). She cites one student's evaluation of the course: "I felt better, relieved of some anxiety and distress. Meeting with the others was very helpful also. It was a supportive atmosphere and gave me a sense of camaraderie and hope" (173). Charon continues to use the parallel chart in her teaching. She has also offered numerous workshops to other health professionals who wish to use this method.

STORYTELLING   Charles M. Anderson, a rhetorician who teaches literature courses to fourth-year medical students at the University of Arkansas for Medical Sciences, began to use oral and written storytelling in his classes when he was "stunned, speechless," by a student who likened Mary Shelley's *Frankenstein* to her experience as a medical student (280). After several years of taping oral stories and reading written ones that he began eliciting from his students, Anderson observed that their stories fell into four main categories. The first three echo themes I have identified in the memoirs of medical education: stories that "signal membership in a specific community"; stories that reflect students' desires to become a part of that community at the same time that they "fear" a loss of personal identity by doing so; and stories in which students recognize the "powerful but unspoken assumptions" about medicine and "ask and address critical questions that normative medical training often marginalizes or silences outright" (282, 284, 288–89).

Anderson's fourth category, which he calls stories of healing, are those in which a student's "pain and confusion . . . open a rhetorical space in which both new and silenced voices can be heard" (290). Anderson describes a process whereby the very act of telling a story—of delving into oneself to find the words that best explain what the experience meant—leads the student to "re-vision" the experience in a way that moves him or her from a sense of emotional isolation to "a more fluid, more narratively able, more socially and professionally integrated self" (291, 281). Stories in this category, Anderson adds, are nearly all written, as the act of writing forces the writer into a "reflective and reflexive . . . space in which the implications of experience" can receive the writer's fullest attention and deliberation (291). Anderson describes writing (as have several of the memoirists I have discussed in previous chapters) as an act that helps them make sense of their experiences and (re)find themselves as physicians. Anderson continues to teach his elective in literature and medicine, and he is frequently invited to teach workshops on personal writing at conferences and medical schools across the country.

These three courses, along with the ones described in the preceding section, share a number of characteristics. They include the use of small groups of students, at least initially, which meet regularly, usually over an extended period of time. Such a format fosters the sharing of stories *if* an atmosphere of trust and safety is developed in the group. All the courses attempt to foster such an environment. The discussions in these groups make purposeful use of self-disclosure. The discussion leaders acknowledge and examine the emotional significance of the students' experiences, even in courses with very pragmatic goals. Carefully structured discussions and assignments convey to students that the faculty regard these expressions of emotion as something more rigorous than a simple venting. Finally, as already mentioned, even though two of Reifler's assignments are now given to the entire class and Charon offers guidelines for teaching the parallel chart,[14] it is nevertheless probable that part of the success of these courses rests upon the faculty member's particular affinity for and belief in the processes of narrative to heighten students' self-awareness.

The courses designed by Reifler, Charon, and Anderson, however, differ from the four courses described more briefly above in their deliberative use of reading and writing. As did those other instructors, they design their writing assignments carefully so that the exercise will lead students to consider particular issues and encourage self-examination. In addition, though, they talk about the tools and process of telling stories, in essence teaching students particular skills in interpretation, whether of another person's story or their own. They are careful and deliberate with their feedback, striving to balance discussion of what the students learn about themselves with explanations of how these narrative skills aid self-discovery. In response to Charon's caution against seeing one's class (or having it be seen) as a therapy session, it is note-worthy that these three teachers pattern both their assignments and the kind of feedback they give so that students may be only as self-disclosing as they want to be. For students who do not come to self-reflection easily or openly, it may be enough to hear other people voicing fears that they also harbor.

The further students venture into narrative, however, the more they stand to gain. Both Charon and Anderson describe the process of writing as a continuous alternation between experiencing emotions and undertaking interpretation, or feeling and thinking. Charon describes narrative as simul-taneously ordering and *dis*ordering: "Narrative is not clean, predictable, or obeisant. . . . Narrative anywhere can make new out of old, creating chaos out of linearity while, subversively, exposing underlying fresh connections among the seemingly unrelated. Not only through its ordering impulses but also through its *disordering* ones, narrative can help one see newly and for the first time something concealed" (219). Anderson's stories that heal are ones in which "the sprawl of [students'] experience can be shaped into . . . coherent, deeply inventive narratives," made possible because in the act of writing "the implications of experience can be invented, discovered, left, picked up again, envisioned, re-visioned and made more permanent and accessible" (290). Both Charon and Anderson describe narrative as nonlinear, which may be counterintuitive to our more familiar notion of stories moving from begin-ning to end, but they refer here to writing as, among other things, a process of selection and scrutiny. In the memoirs of medical education, for example, I pointed out instances in which authors played with chronology, chose to spend more time with some events or people than others, and shifted narrative voice between themselves as author and themselves as character in their own story. In personal writing, an author reencounters every moment of her or his experience—"chaos" for Charon and "sprawl" for Anderson—and emerges with something that is seen, for Charon, "newly and for the first time," and which becomes, for Anderson, "more permanent and accessible."

Anderson's and Charon's articulation of how writing can contribute to a fuller understanding of one's patients and oneself takes narrative beyond an entertaining diversion and gives students skills that they can consciously bring to their clinical work. Indeed, Charon and others have begun using the term *narrative competence* to describe the very pragmatic role narrative can play in a physician's education.[15] The choice of such a term may deliberately reflect medical educators' new attention to competency-based teaching, but it is a valid way to frame this concept. Scholars of narrative and narrative in medicine can thus provide a fuller understanding of how to implement the MSOP's recommendation that medical students "must seek to understand the meaning of patients' stories"[16] and can help educators to understand how inextricable that story is from the story of the student him- or herself.

Narrative competence, however, does not necessarily lead to emotional honesty. Telling a story about oneself or one's patient does position a person to learn about one's beliefs or emotions, but it does not guarantee that such insight will occur. There are several reasons for this, some inherent to the writing process and some to medical education. During the writing process, writers can be so blinded by their emotions or biases that they are incapable of the kind of self-examination described above. Writers may be so persuaded by their own biases that they refuse to consider other options, holding to their position and manipulating the story to serve their point (writing is, after all, also a rhetorical—i.e., persuasive—act). Finally, writing involves the creation of a persona, a characterization of the narrator that may trap writers into stances from which they cannot extricate themselves. Writing contains pitfalls that novice writers may have difficulties avoiding; it also allows outs for writers who would dodge emotional honesty.

The memoirs I have quoted here repeatedly testify to students' ability to learn quickly how to perform well—and to others' expectations—even when they scorn the performance or the person requiring it. We can also deduce from the memoirs that many faculty would be poor teachers of such writing courses should they be implemented generally in medical curricula. In short, achieving true narrative competence, in all that its proponents (myself included) would claim for it, requires emotional honesty of those who would both learn and teach it, bringing me back to the dilemma underscored in so many of these memoirs: undergraduate and graduate medical students crave emotional honesty in their teachers but report it only rarely. How, then, is emotional honesty to be taught? Indeed, *can* it be taught?

The same question has been posed, perennially, in medical education about empathy, compassion, altruism, caring—about all those magical qualities whose roots reside deep in each person's psyche and experience. Certainly medical educators can be urged to sustain and nurture these qualities in their students, but can they be asked to generate a psychological quality that some teachers themselves may not possess in the first place? Periodically, calls are made for screening instruments in the admissions process that will identify such qualities in applicants to medical schools, but no such successful instruments have been developed. Moreover, medicine is hardly the only arena in our society where emotional honesty is needed. Can we expect medical education to take on this moral campaign? Efforts to achieve emotional honesty in all walks of life would be a worthy goal, but I am also wary of any efforts by an institutional body to undertake anything that hints at moral policing. In medical education, however, where patients are an integral part of the physician's learning, the pedagogical stakes are higher.

Personal writing, as Anderson in particular has described it, is an embodied process, in which the act of exploring memory and emotion takes the writer back into the physical feelings of the moment. The physical act of writing as well, whether with pen or keyboard, also engages a person's body, further linking mind and body in this work. For this ability to bring a writer fully to bear on his or her emotional experiences, personal writing is a valuable tool in medical education. It is most valuable, however, when students are made cognizant of the writing process. When writing is accompanied with some instruction in how the writing process and stories "work," narrative becomes not only a way to find community when stories are shared but also a method that students can consciously use on their own. Whatever kinds of personal writing students or residents are asked to produce, however, in whatever setting, some instructor must respond to their writing, to both the emotional content and the narrative tools they use to grapple with their thoughts and feelings. If telling or writing a story is just another assignment, it will quickly be dismissed as busywork and the process of narrative regarded as irrelevant to a physician's work. Teaching with narratives, as with any kind of teaching, is usually most effective when it reflects current experiences and concerns. Reflection groups as part of an ambulatory rotation, parallel charts in an internal medicine clerkship, writing about cadavers in gross anatomy, and a literature elective that includes personal narratives that tie literature to personal experience—all the activities I have described in this chapter bring the narrative work as close to the daily work of the students and residents as possible.

But narratives that foster emotional honesty need not be limited to structured assignments. Although I do believe that learning narrative tools requires some deliberateness, these memoirs of medical education have also demonstrated the value of learning about emotions in personal narratives from their own teachers. These stories occur spontaneously, unplanned, and they respond to an immediate need of an emotionally upset student or resident. These are the stories that say, "I've been there, and I've felt what you're feeling," and, according to the writers of these memoirs, the best of these stories also convey the message that it's not only all right to feel that way now but also that it's all right to feel that way always.

For some teachers in medicine, emotional honesty comes naturally, as it seemed to do for some of the residents that various writers have described in the memoirs. Such conversations do not require training in therapy, do not unleash emotional floodgates, and probably enable students to return to the hospital floor in better shape than had they tried to soldier on (a telling metaphor). Sometimes emotional honesty happens so naturally and quickly that most people probably don't realize what has happened. For example, several years ago I spent a month observing faculty, residents, and medical students on an internal medicine service as they made rounds and met to discuss patients. A regular feature of every day was morning report, the first communal activity of the day, in which students and residents met with one supervisor (usually the department head, residency director, or chief resident) and reviewed the situations of the patients who had been admitted to their service during the night. One morning there was a flurry of discussion about a man who had come into the emergency room in acute distress, with an array of signs and symptoms that pointed to one clear diagnosis. To the annoyance of everyone, someone (never identified) ordered an x-ray, which took valuable time away from emergency treatment—but which revealed an entirely different problem that should not have manifested itself as it had. If that hidden problem had not been accidentally discovered and treated, the man would probably have died within hours. Everyone in the room looked in dismayed disbelief at the x-ray that the radiology resident put onto the screen before them.

After a brief silence, the residency director spoke, directly addressing the junior resident who had been the primary caregiver for this man: "For the next at least one hundred patients who come in looking like this, you are going to waste precious time ordering an x-ray, and you'll never see this again." He paused a few moments. "And you'll have nightmares about this one." The director spoke in a normal tone of voice, not joking, not scolding the resident for all the needless x-rays he would take (or for the x-ray that he hadn't ordered but that saved a man's life). In his tone was the sound of experience, and senior residents around the table nodded, some with a rueful smile, to indicate that they had been in similar situations. He acknowledged how the resident was feeling at that moment—his horror at what had almost happened—and he acknowledged that the horror would follow him for a while and that this was to be expected and was all right, too. The residency director recognized the fears in the young man's story, unspoken in the highly technical language that infuses most medical reporting, and addressed those fears by acknowledging the resident's unique presence in his patient's story and allowing him to imagine himself beyond the shock of the moment. He also told a larger story, of what would inevitably happen to all of them, with a lesson that was taken to heart by everyone in the room.

This residency director, as far as I know, had no instruction in either narrative competence or emotional honesty. He did, however, hear the unstated emotions the resident was experiencing and took the time—less than thirty seconds, hardly a disruption in the busy work of the day—to acknowledge those feelings, establish that such a reaction was entirely normal, and put those feelings within the context of the resident's future experiences. It is an exercise that could be practiced with residents and medical faculty in any of a number of didactic settings that continue to be a part of their ongoing professional development. It depends on physicians' willingness to accept that their job as teachers involves more than imparting knowledge or developing technical and reasoning skills. As accreditation guidelines continue to venture further and further into the language of affect, a place may be found for such training of the teachers of physicians.

The sharp increase in articles that describe and attempt to evaluate courses in medical ethics, health communication, cultural sensitivity or competence, spirituality, integrative medicine, wellness, mindfulness, professionalism, humanities, art—the possibilities have become seemingly endless and increasingly creative—suggests that medical educators are serious in their desire to find new avenues to sustain or foster compassion, empathy, caring, altruism. Given the diverse backgrounds and interests of both students and their teachers, there will never be one curricular magic bullet for addressing emotional honesty or empathy or altruism in medical education. Such a variety of courses and programs, however, is a hopeful sign of a general recognition of the emotional difficulties of becoming a physician, offering a broad spectrum of opportunities for students and teachers to broach these sensitive issues. Although I believe that the skills and discipline required of effective narrative writing provide one of the most efficient routes to self-understanding, I also believe that teachers should teach from their strengths.

Courses that stimulate reflection and emotional honesty, however, can never compensate for an educational environment that is inherently hostile to such exercises. Programs whose main goal is to reduce stress rather than to acknowledge the value of emotions walk a thin line between helping students and placing on their shoulders the burden of adjusting to an unhealthful environment. Students' emotional discomfort with some parts of their medical education, in fact, may be a valuable pedagogical resource. They may be bellwethers for educators and practitioners who have become complacent about their curricula and their professions. If medical education in some part is dysfunctional, it can nevertheless be improved in ways that will serve the humanity of both its graduates and the people who will encounter them as patients. Rethinking the role of emotions in medical education is not an easy task. Emotional honesty is a project for all health professionals, administrators, and professional leaders. But the raw materials are there, in the ideals and motivations of the students who enter colleges of medicine every year and in the stories they tell.

Appendix

The following list of memoirs of medical education includes only the books and blogs that met my strict criteria for inclusion in my study, although I do cite (but seldom more than once or in passing) a few works of fiction and of memoir published after my cutoff date of 2005. I provide this list in particular to provide information about the period covered in each memoir. Although I have argued that the repetition of themes across years makes the actual year of any particular memoir of secondary importance, I know that this information will be of interest to readers.

OVERVIEW OF MEMOIRS CITED

Author	Title of memoir	Date first published	Period covered (approximately)
Baldwin, Emily	Emily Baldwin's Diary	2000–2002	2000–2002
Barton, Brandon	Brandon Barton's Diary	2001–present	2001–present
Collins, Michael	Hot Lights, Cold Steel: Life, Death and Sleepless Nights in a Surgeon's First Years	2005	late 1970s
DasGupta, Sayantani	Her Own Medicine: A Woman's Journey from Student to Doctor	1999	early 1990s
Greenbaum, Dorothy, and Deidre S. Laiken	Lovestrong: A Woman Doctor's True Story of Marriage and Medicine	1984	c. 1972–1978
Greger, Michael	Heart Failure: Diary of a Third Year Medical Student	1999	1997–1998
Harrison, Michelle	A Woman in Residence	1982	late 1970s
Hartman, Brian	Brian Hartman's Diary	2000–present	2000–present

Author	Title of memoir	Date first published	Period covered (approximately)
Hellerstein, David	*Battles of Life and Death*	1986	late 1970s
Hoffmann, Stephen A.	*Under the Ether Dome: A Physician's Apprenticeship at Massachusetts General Hospital*	1986	late 1970s– early 1980s
Horowitz, Steve, and Neil Offen	*Calling Dr. Horowitz*	1977	late 1960s– early 1970s
Huyler, Frank	*The Blood of Strangers*	1999	mid–late 1990s
Imler, Dan	Dan Imler's Diary	2000–present	2000–present
Klass, Perri	*Baby Doctor: A Pediatrician's Training*	1992	late 1980s
	A Not Entirely Benign Procedure: Four Years as a Medical Student	1987	mid 1980s
Klein, Kenneth	*Getting Better: A Medical Student's Story*	1981	early–mid 1970s
Klitzman, Robert	*A Year-Long Night: Tales of a Medical Internship*	1989	early–mid 1980s
Konner, Melvin	*Becoming a Doctor: A Journey of Initiation in Medical School*	1987	early 1980s
LeBaron, Charles	*Gentle Vengeance: An Account of the First Year at Harvard Medical School*	1981	1978
Lee, Mark	Mark Lee's Diary	2001–2004	2001–2004
MacNab, John	*The Education of a Doctor: My First Year on the Wards*	1971	late 1960s

Author	Title of memoir	Date first published	Period covered (approximately)
Maggiore, Ron	Ron Maggiore's Diary	2001–present	2001–present
Marion, Robert	*Learning to Play God: The Coming of Age of a Young Doctor*	1991	mid–late 1980s
Martin, Toni	*How to Survive Medical School*	1983	early–late 1970s
McCarthy, Claire	*Learning How the Heart Beats: The Making of a Pediatrician*	1995	mid 1980s– early 1990s
Miller, Craig	*The Making of a Surgeon in the Twenty-first Century*	2004	mid-late 1990s
Morgan, Elizabeth	*The Making of a Woman Surgeon*	1980	mid 1960s– mid 1970s
Mullan, Fitzhugh	*White Coat, Clenched Fist: The Political Education of an American Physician*	1976	1965–1972
Nolen, William	*The Making of a Surgeon*	1968	mid–late 1950s
Ofri, Danielle	*Singular Intimacies: Becoming a Doctor at Bellevue*	2003	early 1990s
Patterson, Jane, and Linda Madaras	*Woman/Doctor: The Education of Jane Patterson, M.D.*	1983	1963–1968
Rainer, J. Kenyon	*First Do No Harm: Reflections on Becoming a Neurosurgeon*	1987	1976–1979
Reilly, Philip	*To Do No Harm: A Journey through Medical School*	1987	1977–1981

Author	Title of memoir	Date first published	Period covered (approximately)
Rothman, Ellen Lerner	*White Coat: Becoming a Doctor at Harvard Medical School*	1999	1994–1998
Rubin, Theodore Isaac	*Emergency Room Diary*	1972	early 1950s
Sacco, Joseph	*Morphine, Ice Cream, Tears: Tales of a City Hospital*	1989	early 1980s
Taweel, Jamie	Jamie Taweel's Diary	2001–2004	2001–2004
Transue, Emily	*On Call: A Doctor's Days and Nights in Residency*	2004	1997–2001
Vertosick, Frank, Jr.	*When the Air Hits Your Brain*	1996	early–late 1970s
Viscott, David	*The Making of a Psychiatrist*	1972	mid–late 1960s
Whitenton, Kristi	Kristi Whitenton's Diary	2000–2002	2000–2002
X, Doctor	*Intern*	1965	mid 1950s
Young, Audrey	*What Patients Taught Me: A Medical Student's Journey*	2004	mid–late 1990s

Notes

Introduction

1. Williams, *The Autobiography of William Carlos Williams*, 97.
2. Baldwin, Emily Baldwin's Diary (7/21/2002), http://web.archive.org/web/2002121912493/www.studentdoctor.net/med/display.asp?ID=1250.
3. Becker et al., *Boys in White*, see esp. 33–48 and 419–33; and Merton, Reader, and Kendall, *The Student-Physician*, 41.
4. Hafferty, *Into the Valley*, 182, 10. Hafferty credits the concept of resocialization to Brim and Wheeler, *Socialization after Childhood*.
5. Good, *Medicine, Rationality, and Experience*, 65–87.
6. Montgomery, *How Doctors Think*, 4.
7. Ibid., see esp. 202–04.
8. For example, and chronologically: Oliver Bjorksten et al., "Identification of Medical Student Problems"; Lloyd and Gartrell, "A Further Assessment of Medical School Stress"; Mizrahi, "Managing Medical Mistakes"; Rosenberg and Silver, "Medical Student Abuse"; Calkins, Arnold, and Willoughby, "Medical Students' Perceptions of Stress"; Wolf, "Stress, Coping, and Health"; Rosal et al., "A Longitudinal Study of Students' Depression"; Kassebaum and Cutler, "On the Culture of Student Abuse"; Henning, Ey, and Shaw, "Perfectionism"; Bellini, Baime, and Shea, "Variation of Mood and Empathy"; and Cohen et al., "Physiological and Psychological Effects of Delivering Medical News."
9. Again, a brief sampling, chronologically: Michie and Sandhu, "Stress Management"; Stewart et al., "Stress and Vulnerability"; Helmers et al., "Stress and Depressed Mood"; Schor, Pilpel, and Benbassat, "Tolerance of Uncertainty"; Tyssen et al., "Suicidal Ideation"; Kalaça et al., "What Do We Know"; and Kiessling et al., "First Year Medical Students' Perceptions."
10. Malarkey et al., "Influence of Academic Stress"; Whitehouse et al., "Psychosocial and Immune Effects of Self-Hypnosis"; and Marshall et al., "Cytokine Dysregulation Associated with Exam Stress."
11. Rodolfa, Chavoor, and Velasquez, "Counseling Services"; Bell et al., "A Family Day Program"; and Houwink et al., "Help of Third-Year Medical Students."
12. Astin, "Stress Reduction through Mindfulness Meditation"; Novack et al., "Calibrating the Physician"; Pololi et al., "One Year's Experience with a Program to Facilitate Personal and Professional Development"; Donohoe, "Reflections of Physician-Authors on Death"; and Rucker and Shapiro, "Becoming a Physician."

13. Newton et al., "Is There Hardening of the Heart."

14. Shulman, "Knowledge and Teaching" and "Ways of Seeing"; see also "Learning Is at Its Best When There Is Risk."

15. Balint, *The Doctor, His Patient, and the Illness.*

16. The scholarly discussion of stories (and *narrative*, the two terms used variously but often interchangeably) is vast. For two good general overviews, Mitchell, *On Narrative*; and Polkinghorne, *Narrative Knowing and the Human Sciences.* For discussions of story/narrative particularly in nonfiction, see Bruner, *Acts of Meaning*; Folkenflik, ed., *The Culture of Autobiography*; Sturrock, *The Language of Autobiography*; Smith and Watson, eds., *Women, Autobiography, Theory*; and Anderson and McCurdy, eds., *Writing and Healing.*

17. See, for example, Cook, *The Year of the Intern*; Hejinian, *Extreme Remedies*; Ravin, *M.D.*; Schneiderman, *Sea Nymphs by the Hour*; and Shem, *The House of God.*

18. Rush, *The Autobiography of Benjamin Rush*; Blackwell, *Pioneer Work for Women*; Baker, *Fighting for Life*; and Koop, *Koop.*

19. See Poirier, "Ethical Issues in Modern Medical Autobiographies"; Poirier and Borgenicht, "Physician-Authors—Prophets or Profiteers?"; and Poirier, "Role Stress in Medical Education: A Literary Perspective."

20. Koski, "The Autobiography of Medical Education."

21. For an overview of the comments and controversy *The House of God* has raised, see Wear, "*The House of God*: Another Look."

22. Klass, *A Not Entirely Benign Procedure*, 17–19.

23. Baldwin, Emily Baldwin's Diary (5/9/2001), http://web.archive.org/web/2030113154728/www.studentdoctor.net/med/display.asp?ID=653; and Maggiore, Ron Maggiore's Diary (11/8/2001), http://web.archive.org/web/20030113161227/www.studentdoctor.net/med/display.asp?ID=907.

24. *Benét's Reader's Encyclopedia*, 761–62.

25. Ibid., 100–01. For a discussion of the *Bildungsroman* in physicians' writing, see Jones, "Images of Physicians in Literature."

26. Bellah et al., *Habits of the Heart*, 145; esp. 27–51 and 142–63.

27. R. W. B. Lewis, *The American Adam*, esp. 90–155.

28. Ludmerer, *Learning to Heal*, 102–38.

29. For a useful review of many of the popular films about physicians and a collection of critical analyses of representations of medicine and physicians in the media, see, respectively, Dans, *Doctors in the Movies*; and Friedman, ed., *Cultural Sutures.*

30. Camp et al., "Does a Problem-based Medical Curriculum Affect Depression?"; and Toews et al., "Analysis of Stress Levels."

Chapter 1: Voices from the Emergency Room

1. Literary discussion about this phenomenon is called reader-response theory. A good overview of its major proponents and components can be found in Tompkins, ed., *Reader-Response Criticism.*

2. A popular collection of accounts from emergency rooms by physicians across many specialties is Dan Sachs, ed., *Emergency Room*. It includes stories by several of the writers included in this study.
3. Rubin, *Emergency Room Diary*, viii.
4. Ludmerer, *Time to Heal*, 64.
5. Endpoint, http://www.primaryendpoint.com/llp88aa.html?tpl=pe_cv.tpl& section=pe_cv.tpl, last accessed May 5, 2008.
6. Hartman, Brian Hartman's Diary, http://web.archive.org/web/20030219105449/ www.studentdoctor.net/med/brianbio.asp.
7. At the time this book went to press, the status of these diaries was unclear, although at least some of the writers appear to still be posting. The majority of the entries I have quoted have been archived within studentdoctor.net at http://web.archive.org/web/20011217221122/www.studentdoctor.net/med. This address gives access to the eight diaries through 2002. For entries in this archive, I give this URL in the endnotes; in instances where entries have not been archived, I give the address at which I last found the diary entry, although those sites are currently listed as read-only and do not lead me to the document.
8. Baldwin, Emily Baldwin's Diary, http://web.archive.org/web/20021016070744/ www.studentdoctor.net/med/emilybio.asp.
9. Baldwin, entry no. 1170, (5/2/2002), http://web.archive.org/web/20030306144003/ www.studentdoctor.net/med/display.asp?ID=1170.
10. Baldwin, entry no. 1250, (7/21/2002), http://web.archive.org/web/20021219124931/ www.studentdoctor.net/med/display.asp?ID=1250.
11. Baldwin, entry no. 247, (9/20/2000), http://web.archive.org/web/20021130063207/ www.studentdoctor.net/med//display.asp?ID=247; entry no. 284, (10/25/2000), http://web.archive.org/web/20030306143758/www.studentdoctor.net/med/ display.asp?ID=284; and entry no. 1175 (5/6/2002), http://web.archive.org/web/ 20030306143753/www.studentdoctor.net/med/display.asp?ID=1175.
12. See Current residents, Department of Psychiatry, available at University of California, San Francisco, http://psych.ucsf.edu/education.aspx?id=1272, last accessed January 15, 2008.
13. "Introducing Medical Humanities, New Area of Concentration Launched."
14. Baldwin, entry no. 481, (2/2/2001), http://web.archive.org/web/20021130063524/ www.studentdoctor.net/med/display.asp?ID=481.
15. Baldwin, entry no. 481, http://web.archive.org/web/20030331153745/www .studentdoctor.net/med/view_comment.asp?ID=481.

Chapter 2: Water from a Fire Hose

1. Gross anatomy education is the frequent subject of study by scholars both within and outside medicine. See, for example, Hafferty, *Into the Valley*; Carter, *First Cut*; and Giegerich, *Body of Knowledge*.
2. Imler, Dan Imler's Diary (10/27/2000), http://web.archive.org/web/ 20030306144114/ www.studentdoctor.net/med/display1/asp?ID=173.

3. Baldwin, Emily Baldwin's Diary (10/30/2000), http://web.archive.org/web/20021130062905/ www.studentdoctor.net/med/display.asp?ID=288.

4. Imler, Dan Imler's Diary (8/23/2000), http://web.archive.org/web/20030306144318/www.studentdoctor.net/med/display.asp?ID=88.

5. Imler, (9/24/2000), http://web.archive.org/web/20030110201048/www.studentdoctor.net/med//display.asp?ID=133.

6. Imler, (10/23/2000), http://web.archive.org/web/2003036142921/www.studentdoctor.net/med/display.asp?ID=167.

7. Imler, (2/11/2001), http://web.archive.org/web/2003036142633/www.studentdoctor.net/med/display.asp?ID=499.

8. Hartman, Brian Hartman's Diary (10/6/2000), http://web.archive.org/web/20020622225226/www.studentdoctor.net/med/display.asp?ID=150.

9. Baldwin, Emily Baldwin's Diary (10/7/2000), http://web.archive.org/web/20020523082608/www.studentdoctor.net/med/display.asp?ID=265.

10. Klass, *A Not Entirely Benign Procedure*, 34.

11. Hartman, Brian Hartman's Diary (3/25/2001), http://web.archive.org/web/20030424153440/www.studentdoctor.net/med/display.asp?ID=555.

12. Lee, Mark Lee's Diary (1/5/2002), http://web.archive.org/web/20030113162535/www.studentdoctor.net/med/display.asp?ID=989.

13. Imler, Dan Imler's Diary (6/12/2001), http://web.archive.org/web/20030306143526/www.studentdoctor.net/med/display.asp?ID=697.

14. Klass, *A Not Entirely Benign Procedure*, 40.

15. Maggiore, Ron Maggiore's Diary (10/27/2001), http://web.archive.org/web/2003011316103/www.studentdoctor.net/med/display.asp?ID=827.

16. Baldwin, Emily Baldwin's Diary (2/13/2001), http://web.archive.org/web/20021130061325/www.studentdoctor.net/med/display.asp?ID=500.

17. Maggiore, Ron Maggiore's Diary (8/20/2001), http://web.archive.org/web/20030113161625/www.studentdoctor.net/med/display.asp?ID=888.

18. Hartman, Brian Hartman's Diary (11/14/2001), http://web.archive.org/web/20030405051211/www.studentdoctor.net/med/display.asp?ID=803.

19. Imler, Dan Imler's Diary (10/3/2000), http://web.archive.org/web/20030306141542/www.studentdoctor.net/med/display.asp?ID=145.

20. Mullan, *White Coat, Clenched Fist*, 20.

21. Imler, Dan Imler's Diary (12/19/2000), http://web.archive.org/web/20020520101517/www.studentdoctor.net/med/display.asp?ID=370.

22. Klass, *A Not Entirely Benign Procedure*, 62.

23. For more information, see http://www.usmle.org.

24. Baldwin, Emily Baldwin's Diary (6/6/2002), http://web.archive.org/web/20030110203232/www.studentdoctor.net/med/display.asp?ID=1204.

25. For a history of this shift to more outpatient training, see Ludmerer, *A Time to Heal*, 359–61.

26. Taweel, Jamie Taweel's Diary (12/25/2003), http://www.studentdoctor.net/med/display.asp?ID=1599, last accessed 3/31/2004 (I am no longer able to access this address).

27. Lee, Mark Lee's Diary (6/15/2004), http://www.studentdoctor.net/med/display
.asp?ID=1725, last accessed 3/16/2005 (I am no longer able to access this address).

28. Maggiore, Ron Maggiore's Diary (10/3/2002), http://web.archive.org/web/
20030110203758/www.studentdoctor.net/med/display.asp?ID=1309.

29. Maggiore, Ron Maggiore's Diary (7/8/2003), http://www.studentdoctor.net/med
/display.asp?ID=1436, last accessed 8/1/2003 (I am no longer able to access this
address).

30. Imler, Dan Imler's Diary (7/3/2003), http://share.studentdoctor.net/diary/display1
.asp?ID=1434, last accessed 1/15/2008 (I am no longer able to access this address).

31. Hartman, Brian Hartman's Diary (10/20/2003), http://share.studentdoctor.net /
med/display1.asp?ID=1541, last accessed 1/15/2008 (I am no longer able to access
this address).

32. Imler, Dan Imler's Diary (6/25/2004), http://share.studentdoctor.net/diary/
display1.asp?ID=1733, last accessed 1/15/2008 (I am no longer able to access this
address).

Chapter 3: Embodiment

An earlier version of this paper, "Medical Education and the Embodied Physician,"
was published in *Literature and Medicine* 25, no. 2 (Fall 2006): 522–52.

1. MacNab, *The Education of a Doctor*, back jacket design by Lawrence Ratzkin, no
photograph credit given.

2. Damasio, *Descartes' Error*. Scholars in the humanities who draw on studies in
brain and neurology include Felman and Laub, *Testimony*; Herman, *Trauma and
Recovery*; and MacCurdy, "From Trauma to Writing."

3. Barthes, *S/Z*; Brooks, *Body Work*.

4. For a relevant study of medical students' dreams, see Marcus, "Medical Student
Dreams."

5. Mullan, *White Coat, Clenched Fist*, 21.

6. See Bynum and Porter, *Medicine and the Five Senses*; Howell, *Technology in the
Hospital*; and Reiser, *Medicine and the Reign of Technology*.

7. For some early examples, see Heron, *Intensive Care*; and Gino, *The Nurse's Story*.

8. Barton, Brandon Barton's Diary, (9/28/2004), http://share.studentdoctor.net/
diary/display1.asp?ID=2246, last accessed 1/15/08 (I am no longer able to access
this address).

9. Scalia, *The Cutting Edge*, 98–134.

10. Barton, Brandon Barton's Diary (2/4/2002), http://share.studentdoctor.net/med/
display1.asp?ID=1043, last accessed 1/15/08 (I am no longer able to access this
address).

11. Maggiore, Ron Maggiore's Diary, http://web.archive.org/web/20030106104014/
www.studentdoctor.net/med/display.asp?ID=1021; and (2/21/2002), http://web
.archive.org/web/20030309165749/www.studentdoctor.net/med/display.asp?
ID=1070.

12. Morgan, *The Making of a Woman Surgeon*, 120.

13. Klein, *Getting Better*, 137.

14. Sacco, *Morphine, Ice Cream, Tears*, 92.

Chapter 4: Power and Difference

1. Klass, *A Not Entirely Benign Procedure*, 146.

2. Foucault, *The History of Sexuality, Volume I*, see esp. 92–102.

3. Brody, *The Healer's Power*, esp. 36–43.

4. Waitzkin, *The Politics of Medical Encounters*, viii.

5. Scholars across the health sciences, social sciences, and humanities have written extensively in all of these areas. Here, I cite only one landmark publication in each of these areas. For race and ethnicity, Haynes and Smedley, eds., *The Unequal Burden of Cancer*; for gender, Fisher, *In the Patient's Best Interest*; for sexuality, Crimp, ed., *AIDS*; and for disability, Silvers, Wasserman, and Mahowald, *Disability, Difference, Discrimination*.

6. Recent publications in this area include Eiser and Ellis, "Cultural Competence"; Lie, Boker, and Cleveland, "Using the Tool of Assessing Cultural Competence Training"; Gregg and Saha, "Losing Culture on the Way to Competence"; and Hunt, "Clinical Myths of the Cultural 'Other.'"

7. Mullan, *White Coat, Clenched Fist*, 114.

8. X, *Intern*, 113.

9. Patterson and Madaras, *Woman/Doctor*, 93.

10. Sacco, *Morphine, Ice Cream, Tears*, 105.

11. Reilly, *To Do No Harm*, 176–77.

12. Waitzkin, *The Politics of Medical Encounters*, esp. 3–26.

13. Maggiore, Ron Maggiore's Diary (9/4/2002), http://web.archive.org/web/20030110204032/www.studentdoctor.net/med/display/asp?ID=1290.

14. Kenneth M. Ludmerer, *Time to Heal*, 206.

15. Again, there is a rich history of women in medicine from scholars across all disciplines. The most frequently cited books include Lopate, *Women in Medicine*; Morantz-Sanchez, *Sympathy and Science*; and More, *Restoring the Balance*.

16. Morantz-Sanchez, *Sympathy and Science*, 249.

17. "Undergraduate Medical Education."

18. Ibid.

19. Jonas, Etzel, and Barzansky, "Undergraduate Medical Education"; Barzansky, Jonas, and Etzel, "Education Programs in U.S. Medical Schools, 1990–1999"; Barzansky and Etzel, "Education Programs in U.S. Medical Schools, 2001–2002"; and Barzansky and Etzel, "Education Programs in U.S. Medical Schools, 2004–2005."

20. Ibid.

21. Haseltine and Yaw, *Woman Doctor*, 376.

22. Bickel, *Women in Medicine*.

23. Baldwin, Emily Baldwin's Diary (4/16/2001), http://web.archive.org/web/20030113153142/www.studentdoctor.net/med/display.asp?ID=611.

24. Klass, *A Not Entirely Benign Procedure*, 163–66.

25. A sampling of recent articles: Witte, Stratton, and Nora, "Stories from the Field"; Mangus, Hawkins, and Miller, "Prevalence of Harassment and Discrimination"; and Park et al., "Why Are Women Deterred?"

26. These gender-based attributions were initially laid out most fully by Carol Gilligan, *In a Different Voice*. For a useful overview of the reception of Gilligan's theories, see Larrabee, ed., *An Ethic of Care*.

27. Klass, *A Not Entirely Benign Procedure*, 32.

28. The commentary on pimping that is usually cited is Brancati, "The Art of Pimping." See also Wear et al., "Pimping."

29. Klass, *A Not Entirely Benign Procedure*, 63.

30. See Ludmerer, *Time to Heal*, 320–23.

31. "Frequently Asked Questions about the ACGME Common Duty Hour Standards."

32. Accreditation Council for Graduate Medical Education, "The ACGME's Approach to Limit Resident Duty Hours 2006–07."

33. See Ludmerer, *Time to Heal*, 102–13, 318–20.

34. Klass, *A Not Entirely Benign Procedure*, 73–74.

35. See, for example, Parsons et al., "Between Two Worlds"; and Wear et al., "Making Fun of Patients."

Chapter 5: Relationships

1. Dyrbye, Harris, and Rohren, "Early Clinical Experiences."

2. Gilligan, *In a Different Voice*; for a useful overview of the reception of Gilligan's theories, see Larrabee, *An Ethic of Care*.

3. Sherwin, *No Longer Patient*; and Nelson and Nelson, *The Patient in the Family*.

4. There is a large, relevant literature in autobiography studies. See, for example, Bjørklund, *Interpreting the Self*; Rodriguez, *Autobiographical Inscriptions*; and Smith and Watson, eds., *Women, Autobiography, Theory*.

5. Maggiore, Ron Maggiore's Diary, http://www.studentdoctor/net/med/display.asp?ID=1436, last accessed 8/1/2003 (I am no longer able to access this address).

6. Maggiore, Ron Maggiore's Diary (7/10/2001), http://web.archive.org/web/20021107065242/www.studentdoctor.net/med/display.asp?ID=869.

7. Maggiore, Ron Maggiore's Diary (11/7/2004), http://www.studentdoctor.net/diary/display.asp?ID=2408, last accessed 3/16/2005 (I am no longer able to access this address).

8. Imler, Dan Imler's Diary (4/20/2001), http://web.archive.org/web/20030306142243/www.studentdoctor.net/med/display.asp?ID=620.

9. Maggiore, Ron Maggiore's Diary (12/13/2001), http://web.archive.org/web/20030113155308/www.studentdoctor.net/diary/display.asp?ID=951.

10. Lee, Mark Lee's Diary (9/14/2003), http://www.studentdoctor.net/diary/display
.asp?ID=1516, last accessed 3/31/2004 (I am no longer able to access this address).

11. Baldwin, Emily Baldwin's Diary (11/3/2000), http://web.archive.org/web/
20030306143231/www.studentdoctor.net/diary/display.asp?ID=290.

12. Transue, *On Call*, 107–09; and Marion, *Learning to Play God*, 48–49.

13. Burack et al., "Teaching Compassion and Respect."

14. Hartman, Brian Hartman's Diary (12/15/2000), http://web.archive.org/web/
20030313040830/www.studentdoctor.net/med/display.asp?ID=369.

15. Maggiore, Ron Maggiore's Diary (2/5/2002), http://web.archive.org/web/
20030106105826/www.studentdoctor.net/med/display.asp?ID=1062.

16. Klass, *A Not Entirely Benign Procedure*, 33–34.

17. Maggiore, Ron Maggiore's Diary (4/22/2002), http://web.archive.org/web/
20030110200756/www.studentdoctor.net/diary/display.asp?ID=115.

18. Taweel, Jamie Taweel's Diary (9/6/2001), http://web.archive.org/web/
20021102204400/www.studentdoctor.net/diary/display.asp?ID=759.

19. Baldwin, Emily Baldwin's Diary (11/14/2000), http://web.archive.org/web/
20030306141615/www.studentdoctor.net/diary/display.asp?ID=296.

20. Hartman, Brian Hartman's Diary (3/30/2001), http://share.studentdoctor.net/
diary/display1.asp?ID=565, last accessed 1/15/08 (I am no longer able to access
this address).

Conclusion

1. Imler, Dan Imler's Diary (11/5/2003), http://share.studentdoctor.net/med/
display1.asp?ID=1631, last accessed 1/15/08 (I am no longer able to access this
address).

2. For one advocate of such a pedagogy, see Shulman, "Ways of Seeing."

3. Spiro, "What Is Empathy?" 843. Spiro has collected this essay and other, solicited
ones by a variety of medical educators/physicians in *Empathy and the Practice of
Medicine: Beyond Pills and the Scalpel*.

4. "Report of the Working Group on Personal Qualities, Values, and Attitudes,"
177, 178–81.

5. Medical School Objectives Writing Group, "Learning Objectives for Medical
Student Evaluation," 15–16.

6. Accreditation Council on Graduate Medical Education, "Common Program
Requirements."

7. Henry-Tillman et al., "The Medical Student as Patient Navigator."

8. Pololi et al., "One Year's Experience with a Program to Facilitate Personal and
Professional Development," 39, 38.

9. Rucker and Shapiro, "Becoming a Physician," 392.

10. Van Groenou and Bakes, "Art, Chaos, Ethics, and Science," 532.

11. Dyrbye, Thomas, and Shanafelt, "Medical Student Distress," 1617, 1618, and
1619.

12. These three courses are just a sample. For courses that deliberately teach narrative in relation to medicine, besides the journals of academic medicine in which descriptions often appear, there are also two useful collections: Hawkins and McEntyre, eds., *Teaching Literature and Medicine*; and an online collection of course syllabi on the *Literature, Arts, and Medicine Database*, available at http://litmed.med.nyu/Main?action=new.

13. This is a very broad summary of Charon's chapters "Narrative Features of Medicine" and "Close Reading," 39–62 and 107–29.

14. Charon, 159.

15. This term and a call for its cultivation in medical education was also used by Jones, "The Color of the Wallpaper."

16. Medical School Objectives Writing Group, "Learning Objectives for Medical School Evaluation," 16.

Bibliography

Accreditation Council on Graduate Medical Education. "The ACGME's Approach to Limit Resident Duty Hours 2006–07: A Summary of Achievements for the Fourth Year under the Common Requirements." http://www.acgme.org/acWebsite/duty Hours/dh_achieveSum0607.pdf. Last accessed 1/15/08.

———. "Common Program Requirements: General Competencies." http://www .acgme .org/outcome/comp/GeneralCompetenciesStandards221307.pdf. Last accessed 1/15/08.

Alvord, Lori Arviso, and Elizabeth Cohen Van Pelt. *The Scalpel and the Silver Bear: The First Navajo Woman Surgeon Combines Western Medicine and Traditional Healing.* New York: Bantam / Random House, 1999.

Anderson, Charles M. "'Forty acres of cotton waiting to be picked': Medical Students, Storytelling, and the Rhetoric of Healing." *Literature and Medicine* 17, no. 2 (Fall 1988): 280–97.

———, and Marian MacCurdy, eds. *Writing and Healing: Toward an Informed Practice.* Urbana, IL: National Council of Teachers of English, 2000.

Astin, J. A. "Stress Reduction through Mindfulness Meditation: Effects on Psychological Symptomatology, Sense of Control, and Spiritual Experiences." *Psychotherapy and Psychosomatics* 66, no. 2 (1997): 97–106.

Baker, S. Josephine. *Fighting for Life.* New York: Arno, 1974. Originally published 1939.

Baldwin, Emily. Emily Baldwin's Diary. See Medschooldiary.com.

Balint, Michael. *The Doctor, His Patient, and the Illness.* New York: International Univ. Press, 1972.

Barthes, Roland. *S/Z.* Trans. Richard Miller. New York: Hill and Wang, 1974.

Barton, Brandon. Brandon Barton's Diary. See Medschooldiary.com.

Barzansky, Barbara, and Sylvia I. Etzel. "Education Programs in U.S. Medical Schools, 2004–2005." *Journal of the American Medical Association* 292, no. 9 (1 September 2004): 1025–31.

———. "Education Programs in U.S. Medical Schools, 2001–2002." *Journal of the American Medical Association* 288, no. 9 (4 September 2002): 1067–72.

Barzansky, Barbara, Harry S. Jonas, and Sylvia I. Etzel. "Education Programs in U.S. Medical Schools, 1990-1999." *Journal of the American Medical Association* 282, no. 9 (1 September 1999): 840–46.

Becker, Howard S., Blanche Geer, Everett C. Hughes, and Anselm L. Strauss. *Boys in White: Student Culture in Medical School.* Chicago: Univ. of Chicago Press, 1961.

Bell, Mary A., Paula S. Smith, James J. Brokaw, and Herbert E. Cushing. "A Family Day Program Enhances Knowledge about Medical School Culture and Necessary

Supports." *BMC Medical Education* 4, no. 3 (2004). http://www.biomedcentral.com /1472–6920/4/3.

Bellah, Robert H., Richard Madsen, William M. Sullivan, Ann Swidler, and Steven M. Tipton. *Habits of the Heart: Individualism and Commitment in American Life.* Berkeley: Univ. of California Press, 1985.

Bellini, Lisa M., Michael Baime, and Judy A. Shea. "Variation of Mood and Empathy during Internship." *Journal of the American Medical Association* 287, no. 23 (19 June 2002): 3143–46.

Benét's Reader's Encyclopedia. 3d ed. New York: Harper and Row, 1987.

Bickel, Janet W. *Women in Medicine: Getting In, Growing, and Advancing.* Thousand Oaks, CA: Sage, 2000.

Biro, David. *One Hundred Days: My Unexpected Journey from Doctor to Patient.* New York: Pantheon, 2000.

Bjørklund, Diane. *Interpreting the Self: Two Hundred Years of American Autobiography.* Chicago: Univ. of Chicago Press, 1998.

Bjorksten, Oliver, Susan Sutherland, Clinton Miller, and Thomas Stewart. "Identification of Medical Student Problems and Comparison with Those of Other Students." *Journal of Medical Education* 58 (October 1983): 759–67.

Blackwell, Elizabeth. *Pioneer Work in Opening the Medical Profession to Women.* New York: Longmans, Green, 1895. Reprinted as *Opening the Medical Profession to Women,* New York: Schocken Books, 1977.

Brancati, Frederick L. "The Art of Pimping." *Journal of the American Medical Association* 262, no. 1 (7 July 1989): 89–90.

Brim, Orville G., Jr., and Stanton Wheeler. *Socialization after Childhood: Two Essays.* New York: John Wiley, 1966.

Brody, Howard. *The Healer's Power.* New Haven: Yale Univ. Press, 1992.

Brooks, Peter. *Body Work: Objects of Desire in Modern Narrative.* Cambridge: Harvard Univ. Press, 1993.

Bruner, Jerome. *Acts of Meaning.* Cambridge: Harvard Univ. Press, 1990.

Bryant, Daniel C. "Roster of Physician Writers." Available at http://library.med.nyu .edu/library/eresources/featurecollections/bryant/roster.html.

Burack, Jeffrey H., David M. Irby, Jan D. Carline, Richard K. Root, and Eric B. Larson. "Teaching Compassion and Respect." *Journal of General Internal Medicine* 14, no. 1 (January 1999): 49–55.

Butler, Judith. *Bodies That Matter: On the Discursive Limits of "Sex."* New York: Routledge, 1993.

Bynum, W. F., and Roy Porter, eds. *Medicine and the Five Senses.* Cambridge: Cambridge Univ. Press, 1993.

Calkins, E. Virginia, Louise Arnold, and T. Lee Willoughby. "Medical Students' Perceptions of Stress: Gender and Ethnic Considerations." *Academic Medicine* 69, no. 10 (October supplement 1994): S22–24.

Camp, D. Lawrence, Merris A. Hollingsworth, Daniel J. Zaccaro, Liza D. Cariago-Lo, and Boyd F. Richards. "Does a Problem-based Learning Curriculum Affect

Depression in Medical Students?" *Academic Medicine* 69, no. 10 (October supplement 1994): S25–27.

Campo, Rafael. *The Poetry of Healing: A Doctor's Education in Empathy, Identity, and Desire.* New York: W. W. Norton, 1997.

Carson, Ben, and Greg Lewis. *The Big Picture.* Grand Rapids, MI: Zondervan, 2000.

———, with Cecil Murphey. *Gifted Hands: The Ben Carson Story.* Grand Rapids, MI: Zondervan, 1990.

Carter, Albert Howard, III. *First Cut: A Season in the Human Anatomy Lab.* New York: Picador, 1997.

Charon, Rita. *Narrative Medicine: Honoring the Stories of Illness.* New York: Oxford Univ. Press, 2006.

Chen, Pauline W. *Final Exam: A Surgeon's Reflections on Mortality.* New York: Alfred A. Knopf, 2007.

Cohen, Lorenzo, Walter F. Balie, Evelyn Henninger, Sandeep K. Agarwal, Renato Lenzi, Janet Sterner, and Gailen D. Marshall. "Physiological and Psychological Effects of Delivering Medical News Using a Simulated Physician-Patient Scenario." *Journal of Behavioral Medicine* 26, no. 5 (October 2003): 459–71.

Collins, Michael J. *Hot Lights, Cold Steel: Life, Death, and Sleepless Nights in a Surgeon's First Years.* New York: St. Martin's, 2005.

Cook, Robin. *The Year of the Intern.* New York: A Signet Book / New American Library, 1972.

Coulehan, John L. "Tenderness and Steadiness: Emotions in Medical Practice." *Literature and Medicine* 14, no. 2 (Fall 1995): 222–36.

Crichton, Michael. *Five Patients: The Hospital Explained.* New York: Alfred A. Knopf, 1970.

Crimp, Douglas, ed. *AIDS: Cultural Analysis, Cultural Activism.* 1987; rpt. Cambridge, MA: MIT Press, 1988.

Damasio, Antonio. *Descartes' Error: Emotion, Reason, and the Human Brain.* New York: G. P. Putnam's Sons, 1994.

Dans, Peter E. *Doctors in the Movies.* Bloomington, IL: Medi-Ed Press, 2000.

DasGupta, Sayantani. *Her Own Medicine: A Woman's Journey from Student to Doctor.* New York: Fawcett Gold Medal, 1999.

Dawson, Patricia L. *Forged by the Knife: The Experience of Surgical Residency from the Perspective of a Woman of Color.* Greensboro, NC: Open Hand Publishing, 1999.

Donohoe, Martin. "Reflections of Physician-Authors on Death: Literary Selections Appropriate for Teaching Rounds." *Journal of Palliative Medicine* 5, no. 6 (December 2002): 843–48.

Dooley, Thomas A. *The Night They Burned the Mountain.* New York: Farrar, Straus, and Cudahy, 1960.

Dyrbye, Lisolette N., Ilene Harris, and Charles H. Rohren. "Early Clinical Experiences from Students' Perspectives: A Qualitative Study of Narratives." *Academic Medicine* 82, no. 10 (October 2007): 979–88.

Dyrbye, Lisolette N., Matthew R. Thomas, and Tait D. Shanafelt. "Medical Student Distress: Causes, Consequences, and Proposed Solutions." *Mayo Clinic Proceedings* 80, no. 12 (December 2005): 1613–22.

Eakin, Paul John. *How Our Lives Become Stories: Making Selves.* Ithaca: Cornell Univ. Press, 1999.

Eiser, Arnold R., and Glenn Ellis. "Cultural Competence and the African American Experience with Health Care: The Case for Specific Content in Cultural-Competency Education." *Academic Medicine* 82, no. 2 (February 2007): 176–83.

Felman, Shoshana, and Dori Laub. *Testimony: Crises of Witnessing in Literature, Psycho-analysis, and History.* New York: Routledge, 1992.

Fisher, Sue. *In the Patient's Best Interest: Women and the Politics of Medical Decisions.* New Brunswick: Rutgers Univ. Press, 1986.

Folkenflik, Robert, ed. *The Culture of Autobiography: Constructions of Self-Representation.* Stanford: Stanford Univ. Press, 1993.

Foucault, Michel. *The Birth of the Clinic: An Archeology of Medical Perception.* Trans. A. M. Sheridan Smith. New York: Pantheon Books, 1973. Originally published in French in 1963.

———. *The History of Sexuality, Volume I: An Introduction.* Trans. Robert Hurley. New York: New Vintage Books / Random House, 1980. Originally published in French in 1976.

"Frequently Asked Questions about the ACGME Common Duty Hour Standards." http://www.acgme.org/acWebsite/dutyHours/dh_faqs.pdf. Last accessed 1/15/08.

Friedman, Lester D., ed. *Cultural Sutures: Medicine and Media.* Durham: Duke Univ. Press, 2004.

Gawande, Atul. *Complications: A Surgeon's Notes on an Imperfect Science.* New York: Metropolitan Books / Henry Holt, 2002.

Giegerich, Steve. *Body of Knowledge: One Semester of Gross Anatomy, the Gateway to Becoming a Doctor.* New York: Simon and Schuster / Touchstone Books, 2001.

Gilligan, Carol. *In a Different Voice: Psychological Theory and Women's Development.* Cambridge: Harvard Univ. Press, 1982.

Gino, Carol. *The Nurse's Story.* New York: Simon and Schuster, 1982.

Gonzalez-Crussi, F. *Notes of an Anatomist.* San Diego: Harcourt Brace Jovanovich, 1985.

Good, Byron. *Medicine, Rationality, and Experience: An Anthropological Perspective.* Cambridge: Cambridge Univ. Press, 1994.

Greenbaum, Dorothy, and Deidre S. Laiken. *Lovestrong: A Woman Doctor's True Story of Marriage and Medicine.* New York: Signet Books / New American Library, 1984.

Greer, Pedro José, with Liz Balmaseda. *Waking Up in America: How One Doctor Brings Hope to Those Who Need It Most.* New York: Touchstone / Simon and Schuster, 1999.

Greger, Michael. *Heart Failure: Diary of a Third-Year Medical Student.* Jamaica Plain, MA: Michael Greger, 1999.

Gregg, Jessica, and Samnath Saha. "Losing Culture on the Way to Competence: The Use and Misuse of Culture in Medical Education." *Academic Medicine* 81, no. 6 (June 2006): 542–47.

Groopman, Jerome E. *How Doctors Think*. New York: Houghton Mifflin, 2007.

Hafferty, Frederic W. *Into the Valley: Death and the Socialization of Medical Students*. New Haven: Yale Univ. Press, 1991.

Harrison, Michelle. *A Woman in Residence*. New York: Random House, 1982.

Hartman, Brian. Brian Hartman's Diary. See Medschooldiary.com.

Haseltine, Florence, and Yvonne Yaw. *Woman Doctor*. New York: Ballantine Books, 1976.

Hawkins, Anne Hunsaker, and Marilyn Chandler McEntyre, eds. *Teaching Literature and Medicine*. New York: Modern Language Association, 2000.

Haynes, M. Alfred, and Brian D. Smedley, eds. *The Unequal Burden of Cancer: An Assessment of NIH Research and Programs for Ethnic Minorities and the Medically Underserved*. Committee on Cancer Research among Minorities and the Medically Underserved, Health Sciences Policy Program, Health Sciences Section, Institute of Medicine. Washington, DC: National Academy Press, 1999.

Hejinian, John. *Extreme Remedies*. New York: St. Martin's, 1994.

Hellerstein, David. *Battles of Life and Death*. New York: Warner Books, 1986.

Helmers, Karin F., Deborah Danoff, Yvonne Steinert, Marco Leyton, and Simon H. Young. "Stress and Depressed Mood in Medical Students, Law Students, and Graduate Students." *Academic Medicine* 72, no. 8 (August 1997): 708–14.

Henning, Kris, Sydney Ey, and Darlene Shaw. "Perfectionism, the Imposter Phenomenon, and Psychological Adjustment in Medical, Dental, Nursing, and Pharmacy Students." *Medical Education* 32, no. 5 (September 1998): 456–64.

Henry-Tillman, Ronda, Linda A. Deloney, Mildred Savidge, C. James Graham, and V. Suzanne Klimberg. "The Medical Student as Patient Navigator as an Approach to Teaching Empathy." *American Journal of Surgical Education* 183, no. 6 (June 2002): 569–62.

Herman, Judith. *Trauma and Recovery*. New York: Basic Books, 1992.

Heron, Echo. *Intensive Care*. New York: Atheneum, 1987.

Hilfiker, David. *Not All of Us Are Saints: A Doctor's Journey with the Poor*. New York: Hill and Wang, 1994.

Hoffmann, Stephen A. *Under the Ether Dome: A Physician's Apprenticeship at Massachusetts General Hospital*. New York: Charles Scribner's Sons, 1986.

Horowitz, Steve, and Neil Offen. *Calling Dr. Horowitz*. New York: William Morrow, 1997.

Houwink, Aletta P., Anil N. Kurup, Joshua P. Kollars, Catharine A. Kral Kollars, Stephen W. Carmichael, and Wojciech Pawlina. "Help of Third-Year Medical Students Decreases First-Year Medical Students' Negative Psychological Reactions on the First Day of Gross Anatomy Dissection." *Clinical Anatomy* 17 (2004): 328–33.

Howell, Joel D. *Technology in the Hospital*. Baltimore: Johns Hopkins Univ. Press, 1995.

Hunt, Linda M. "Clinical Myths of the Cultural 'Other': Implications for Latino Patient Care." *Academic Medicine* 80, no. 10 (October 2005): 918–24.

Hunter, Kathryn Montgomery. *Doctors' Stories: The Narrative Structure of Medical Knowledge*. Princeton: Princeton Univ. Press, 1991.

Huyler, Frank. *The Blood of Strangers*. New York: Owl Books / Henry Holt, 1999.

Iezzoni, Lisa I. *When Walking Fails: Mobility Problems of Adults with Chronic Conditions*. Berkeley: Univ. of California Press, 2003.

Imler, Daniel. Daniel Imler's Diary. See Medschooldiary.com.

"Introducing Medical Humanities, New Area of Concentration Launched." UCSF School of Medicine. News, May 17, 2004. http://medschool.ucsf.edu/news/ features/education/051704_Humanities AoC.aspx. Last accessed 1/15/2008.

Jonas, Harry S., Sylvia I. Etzel, and Barbara Barzansky. "Undergraduate Medical Education." *Journal of the American Medical Association* 264, no. 7 (15 August 1990): 801–09.

Jones, Anne Hudson. "The Color of the Wallpaper: Training for Medical Ethics." In *Stories Matter: The Role of Narrative in Medical Ethics*, 160–67. Rita Charon and Martha Montello, eds. New York: Routledge, 2002.

———. "Images of Physicians in Literature: Medical Bildungsromans." *Lancet* 348 (1996): 734–36.

Kalaça, Sibel, Özlem Sarikaya, Devrim Keklik, and M. Ali Gülpínar. "What Do We Know about the Anxieties of New Clinical Students?" Letter to the editor. *Medical Education* 37, no. 4 (April 2003): 390.

Kaplan, Jonathan. *The Dressing Station: A Surgeon's Chronicle of War and Medicine*. New York: Grove, 2001.

Kassebaum, Donald G., and Ellen R. Cutler. "On the Culture of Student Abuse in Medical School." *Academic Medicine* 73, no. 11 (November 1998): 1149–58.

Kiessling, Claudia, Benjamin Schubert, Dieter Scheffner, and Walter Burger. "First Year Medical Students' Perceptions of Stress and Support: A Comparison between Reformed and Traditional Track Curricula." *Medical Education* 38, no. 5 (May 2004): 504–09.

Klass, Perri. *Baby Doctor*. New York: Random House, 1992.

———. *A Not Entirely Benign Procedure: Four Years as a Medical Student*. New York: G. P. Putnam's Sons, 1987.

Klein, Kenneth. *Getting Better: A Medical Student's Story*. Boston: Little, Brown, 1981.

Klitzman, Robert. *A Year-Long Night: Tales of a Medical Internship*. New York: Penguin Books, 1989.

Konner, Melvin. *Becoming a Doctor: A Journey of Initiation in Medical School*. New York: Elisabeth Sifton Books / Viking, 1987.

Koop, C. Everett. *Koop*. New York: Random House, 1991.

Koski, Cheryl A. "The Autobiography of Medical Education: Anatomy of a Genre." PhD diss., University of Tennessee, 2002.

Lakoff, George, and Mark Johnson. *Metaphors We Live By*. Chicago: Univ. of Chicago Press, 1980.

Lam, Vincent. *Bloodletting and Miraculous Cures*. Canada: Anchor Canada, 2005.

Larrabee, Mary Jeanne, ed. *An Ethic of Care: Feminist and Interdisciplinary Perspectives*. New York: Routledge, 1993.

"Learning Is Best When There Is Risk." News release, March 3, 2006. Available at http//my.brandeis.edu/news/item?news%5item%fid=104486&show%5frelease %5date=1.

LeBaron, Charles. *Gentle Vengeance: An Account of the First Year at Harvard Medical School.* New York: Richard Marek, 1981.

Lee, Mark. Mark Lee's Diary. See Medschooldiary.com.

Lewis, R. W. B. *The American Adam: Innocence, Tragedy, and Tradition in the Nineteenth Century.* Chicago: Univ. of Chicago Press, 1955.

Lewis, Sinclair. *Arrowsmith.* New York: Harcourt, Brace, 1925.

Lie, Désirée, John Boker, and Ella Cleveland. "Using the Tool of Assessing Cultural Competence Training (TACCT) to Measure Faculty and Medical Students' Perceptions of Cultural Competence Instruction in the First Three Years of the Curriculum." *Academic Medicine* 81, no. 6 (June 2006): 557–64.

Literature, Arts, and Medicine Database. Available at http://litmed.med.nyu/Main? action=new.

Lloyd, Camille, and Nanette K. Gartrell. "A Further Assessment of Medical School Stress." *Journal of Medical Education* 58 (December 1983): 964–67.

Lopate, Carol. *Women in Medicine.* Baltimore: Johns Hopkins Univ. Press, 1968.

Ludmerer, Kenneth M. *Learning to Heal: The Development of American Medical Education.* New York: Basic Books, 1985.

———. *Time to Heal: American Medical Education from the Turn of the Century to the Era of Managed Care.* New York: Oxford Univ. Press, 1999.

MacCurdy, Marian. "From Trauma to Writing: A Theoretical Model for Practical Use." In *Writing and Healing: Toward an Informed Practice,* 158–200. Charles M. Anderson and Marian MacCurdy, eds. Urbana, IL: National Council of Teachers of English, 2000.

MacNab, John. *The Education of a Doctor: My First Year on the Wards.* New York: Simon and Schuster, 1971.

Maggiore, Ron. Ron Maggiore's Diary. See Medschooldiary.com.

Malarkey, W. B., D. K. Pearl, L. M. Demers, J. K. Kiecolt-Glaser, and R. Glaser. "Influence of Academic Stress and Season on 24-hour Mean Concentrations of ACTH, Cortisol, and Beta-endorphin." *Psychoneuroendocrinology* 20, no. 5 (1995): 499–508.

Mangus, R. S., C. E. Hawkins, and M. H. Miller. "Prevalence of Harassment and Discrimination among 1996 Medical School Graduates: A Survey of Eight U.S. Schools." *Journal of the American Medical Association* 280, no. 9 (2 September 1998): 851–54.

Marcus, Eric R. "Medical Student Dreams about Medical School: The Unconscious Developmental Process of Becoming a Physician." *International Journal of Psychoanalysis* 84 (2003): 367–86.

Marion, Robert. *Learning to Play God: The Coming of Age of a Young Doctor.* Reading, MA: Addison-Wesley, 1991.

Marshall, G. D., Jr., S. K. Agarwal, C. Lloyd, L. Cohen, E. M. Henninger, and G. J. Morris. "Cytokine Dysregulation Associated with Exam Stress in Healthy Medical Students." *Brain Behavior and Immunity* 12, no. 4 (December 1998): 297–30.

Martin, Toni. *How to Survive Medical School.* New York: Penguin, 1984. Originally published New York: Holt, Rinehart, and Winston, 1983.

McCarthy, Claire. *Learning How the Heart Beats: The Making of a Pediatrician*. New York: Viking, 1995.

Medical School Objectives Writing Group. "Learning Objectives for Medical Student Evaluation—Guidelines for Medical Schools: Report 1 of the Medical School Objectives Project." *Academic Medicine* 74, no. 1 (January 1999): 13–18.

Medschooldiary.com. Available at http://web.archive.org/web/20011217221122/www.studentdoctor.net.

Merton, Robert K., George G. Reader, and Patricia L. Kendall, eds. *The Student-Physician*. Cambridge: Harvard Univ. Press, 1957.

Michie, S., and S. Sandhu. "Stress Management for Clinical Medical Students." *Medical Education* 28, no. 6 (November 1994): 528–33.

Miller, Craig A. *The Making of a Surgeon in the Twenty-first Century*. Nevada City, CA: Blue Dolphin, 2004.

Miller, Jean Baker. *Toward a New Psychology of Women*. Boston: Beacon, 1976.

Mitchell, W. J. T. *On Narrative*. Chicago: Univ. of Chicago Press, 1981.

Mizrahi, Terry. "Managing Medical Mistakes: Ideology, Insularity, and Accountability among Internists-in-Training." *Social Science and Medicine* 19, no. 2 (1984): 135–46.

Montgomery, Kathryn. *How Doctors Think: Clinical Judgment and the Practice of Medicine*. Oxford: Oxford Univ. Press, 2006.

Morantz-Sanchez, Regina Markell. *Sympathy and Science: Women Physicians in American Medicine*. New York: Oxford Univ. Press, 1985.

More, Ellen S. *Restoring the Balance: Women Physicians and the Profession of Medicine, 1850–1995*. Cambridge: Harvard Univ. Press, 1999.

Morgan, Elizabeth. *The Making of a Woman Surgeon*. New York: G. P. Putnam's Sons, 1980.

Mullan, Fitzhugh. *Vital Signs: A Young Doctor's Struggle with Cancer*. New York: Farrar, Straus, and Giroux, 1975.

———. *White Coat, Clenched Fist: The Political Education of an American Physician*. New York: Macmillan, 1976.

Nelson, Hilde Lindemann, and James Lindemann Nelson. *The Patient in the Family: An Ethics of Patients and Families*. New York: Routledge, 1995.

Newton, Bruce W., Laurie Barber, James Clardy, Elton Cleveland, and Patricia O'Sullivan. "Is There Hardening of the Heart during Medical School?" *Academic Medicine* 83, no. 3 (March 2008): 244–49.

Nolen, William. *The Making of a Surgeon*. New York: Random House, 1968.

Novack, Dennis H., Anthony L. Suchman, William Clark, Ronald M. Epstein, Eva Najberg, and Craig Kaplan. "Calibrating the Physician: Personal Awareness and Effective Patient Care." *Journal of the American Medical Association* 278, no. 6 (13 August 1997): 502–09.

Nuland, Sherwin B. *Lost in America: A Journey with My Father*. New York: Alfred A. Knopf, 2003.

Ofri, Danielle. *Singular Intimacies: Becoming a Doctor at Bellevue*. Boston: Beacon, 2003.

Osborne, Claudia. *Over My Head: A Doctor's Own Story of Head Injury from the Inside Looking Out*. Kansas City, MO: Andrews McMeel Publishing, 1998.

Park, Jason, Sam Minor, Rebecca Anne Taylor, Elena Vikus, and Don Polnaru. "Why Are Women Deterred from General Surgery Training?" *American Journal of Surgery* 190, no. 1 (July 2005): 141–46.

Parrish, John A. *12, 20, and 5: A Doctor's Year in Vietnam*. New York: E. P. Dutton, 1972.

Parsons, Genevieve Noone, Sara M. Kinsman, Charles L. Bosk, Pamela Sankar, and Peter A. Ubel. "Between Two Worlds: Medical Student Perceptions of Humor and Slang in the Hospital Setting." *Journal of General Internal Medicine* 16, no. 8 (August 2001): 544–49.

Patterson, Jane, and Lynda Madaras. *Woman/Doctor: The Education of Jane Patterson, M.D.* New York: Avon, 1983.

Pilger, John, ed. *Tell Me No Lies: Investigative Journalism That Changed the World*. New York: Thunder's Mouth Press, 2005.

Poirier, Suzanne. "Ethical Issues in Modern Medical Autobiographies." *Perspectives in Biology and Medicine* 30, no. 2 (Winter 1987): 278–89.

———. "Role Stress in Medical Education: A Literary Perspective." *Journal of the American Medical Women's Association* 41, no. 3 (May–June 1986): 82–86.

———, and Lou Borgenicht. "Physician-Authors—Prophets or Profiteers?" Book review. *New England Journal of Medicine* 325 (18 July 1991): 212–14.

Polkinghorne, Donald E. *Narrative Knowing and the Human Sciences*. Albany: State Univ. of New York Press, 1988.

Pololi, Linda, Richard M. Frankel, Maria Clay, and Ann C. Jobe. "One Year's Experience with a Program to Facilitate Personal and Professional Development in Medical Students Using Reflective Groups." *Education for Health* 14, no. 1 (2001): 36–49.

Protess, David L., Fay Lomax Cook, Jack C. Doppelt, James S. Ettema, Margaret T. Gordon, Donna R. Leff, and Peter Miller. *The Journalism of Outrage: Investigative Reporting and Agenda Building in America*. New York: Guilford Press, 1991.

Rainer, J. Kenyon. *First Do No Harm: Reflections on Becoming a Brain Surgeon*. New York: Villard Books, 1987.

Ravin, Neil. *M.D.* N.p.: Delacorte / Seymour Lawrence, 1981.

Reifler, Douglas R. "'I actually don't mind the bone saw': Narratives of Gross Anatomy." *Literature and Medicine* 15, no. 2 (Fall 1996): 183–99.

Reilly, Philip. *To Do No Harm: A Journey through Medical School*. Dover, MA: Auburn House, 1987.

Reiser, Stanley Joel. *Medicine and the Reign of Technology*. Cambridge: Cambridge Univ. Press, 1978.

"Report of the Working Group on Personal Qualities." *Physicians for the Twenty-First Century: Report of the Project Panel on the General Professional Education of the Physician and College Preparation for Medicine. Journal of Medical Education* 59, no. 11, part 2 (November 1984): 177–89.

Rodolfa, Emil, Shelley Chavoor, and Jo Velasquez. "Counseling Services at the University of California, Davis: Helping Medical Students Cope." *Journal of the American Medical Association* 274, no. 17 (1 November 1995): 1396–97.

Rodriguez, Barbara. *Autobiographical Inscriptions: Form, Person, and the American Woman Writer of Color*. New York: Oxford Univ. Press, 1999.

Rosal, Milagros C., Ira S. Ockene, Judith K. Ockene, Susan V. Barrett, Yunsheng Ma, and James R. Herbert. "A Longitudinal Study of Students' Depression in One Medical School." *Academic Medicine* 72, no. 6 (June 1997): 542–46.

Rosenberg, Donna A., and Henry K. Silver. "Medical Student Abuse: An Unnecessary and Preventable Cause of Stress." *Journal of the American Medical Association* 251 (1984): 739–42.

Rothman, Ellen Lerner. *White Coat: Becoming a Doctor at Harvard Medical School*. New York: Perennial / HarperCollins, 1999.

Rubin, Theodore Isaac. *Alive and Fat and Thinning in America*. New York: Coward, McCann, and Geoghegan, 1978.

———. *The Angry Book*. New York: Macmillan, 1969.

———. *Emergency Room Diary*. New York: Grosset and Dunlap / National General, 1972.

———. *Forever Thin*. New York: B. Geis Associates, 1970.

———. *Lisa and David; Jordi; Little Raphie and the Creature*. New York: Forge / Tom Doherty Associates, 1998. Originally published 1960, 1961.

———. *Platzo and the Mexican Pony Rider*. New York: Trident, 1965.

———. *Reflections in a Goldfish Tank*. New York: Coward, McCann, and Geohegan, 1977.

———. *The Thin Book by a Formerly Fat Psychiatrist*. New York: Trident, 1966.

Rucker, Lloyd, and Johanna Shapiro. "Becoming a Physician: Students' Creative Projects in a Third-year IM Clerkship." *Academic Medicine* 78, no. 4 (April 2003): 391–97.

Rush, Benjamin. *The Autobiography of Benjamin Rush*. Princeton: Princeton Univ. Press, 1948. Originally written 1800.

Sacco, Joseph. *Morphine, Ice Cream, Tears: Tales of a City Hospital*. New York: Pinnacle Books / Windsor, 1989.

Sachs, Dan, ed. *Emergency Room: Lives Saved and Lost: Doctors Tell Their Stories*. New York: Little, Brown, 1996.

Sacks, Oliver. *A Leg to Stand On*. London: Picador / Pan Books, 1984.

———. *The Man Who Mistook His Wife for a Hat and Other Clinical Tales*. New York: Summit Books, 1985.

Salber, Eva. *The Mind Is Not the Heart*. Durham: Duke Univ. Press, 1989.

Scalia, Joni Lynn. *The Cutting Edge*. New York: Berkley Books, 1983. Originally published New York: McGraw-Hill, 1978.

Scannell, Kate. *Death of the Good Doctor: Lessons from the Heart of the AIDS Epidemic*. San Francisco: Cleis, 1999.

Schneiderman, L. J. *Sea Nymphs by the Hour*. New York: Bobbs Merrill, 1972. Currently available, Authors Guild Backprint.com Edition (Lincoln, NE: iUniverse .com, 2000).

Schön, Donald. *Educating the Reflective Practitioner: Toward a New Design for Teaching and Learning in the Professions*. San Francisco: Josey-Bass, 1987.

Schor, Razia, Dina Pilpel, and Jochanan Benbassat. "Tolerance of Uncertainty of Medical Students and Practicing Physicians." *Medical Care* 38, no. 3 (March 2000): 272–80.

Selwyn, Peter. *Surviving the Fall: The Personal Journey of an AIDS Doctor.* New Haven: Yale Univ. Press, 1998.

Selzer, Richard. *Raising the Dead.* New York: White Books / Viking, 1994.

Shem, Samuel. *The House of God.* New York: Richard Marek, 1978.

Sherwin, Susan. *No Longer Patient: Feminist Ethics and Health Care.* Philadelphia: Temple Univ. Press, 1992.

Shulman, Lee. "Knowledge and Teaching: Foundations of the New Reform." *Harvard Educational Review* 57, no. 1 (1987): 1–22.

———. "Ways of Seeing, Ways of Knowing, Ways of Teaching, Ways of Learning about Teaching." *Journal of Curriculum Studies* 28 (September–October 1992): 393–96.

Silvers, Anita, David Wasserman, and Mary B. Mahowald. *Disability, Difference, Discrimination: Perspectives on Justice in Bioethics and Public Policy.* Lanham, MD: Rowman and Littlefield, 1998.

Smith, Sidonie, and Julia Watson, eds. *Women, Autobiography, Theory: A Reader.* Madison: Univ. of Wisconsin Press, 1998.

Spiro, Howard, ed. *Empathy and the Practice of Medicine: Beyond Pills and the Scalpel.* New Haven: Yale Univ. Press, 1993.

———. "What Is Empathy and Can It Be Taught?" *Annals of Internal Medicine* 116, no. 10 (15 May 1992): 843–46.

Stewart, S. M., C. Betson, I. Marshall, C. M. Wong, P. W. H. Lee, and T. H. Lam. "Stress and Vulnerability in Medical Students." *Medical Education* 29 (1995): 119–27.

Student Doctor Network. Available at http://www.studentdoctor.net.

Sturrock, John. *The Language of Autobiography: Studies in the First Person Singular.* Cambridge: Cambridge Univ. Press, 1993.

Takakuwa, Kevin M., Nick Rubashkin, and Karen E. Herzig, eds. *What I Learned in Medical School: Personal Stories of Young Doctors.* Berkeley: Univ. of California Press, 2004.

Taweel, Jamie. Jamie Taweel's Diary. See Medschooldiary.com.

Toews, John A., Jocelyn M. Lockyer, Deborah J. G. Dobson, Elizabeth Simpson, A. Keith W. Brownell, Fraser Brenneis, Kathleen M. MacPherson, and Gerald S. Cohen. "Analysis of Stress Levels among Medical Students, Residents, and Graduate Students at Four Canadian Schools of Medicine." *Academic Medicine* 72, no. 11 (November 1997): 997–1002.

Tompkins, Jane P., ed. *Reader-Response Criticism: From Formalism to Post-Structuralism.* Baltimore: Johns Hopkins Univ. Press, 1980.

Transue, Emily. *On Call: A Doctor's Days and Nights in Residency.* New York: St. Martin's, 2004.

Turner, Victor. *Dramas, Fields, and Metaphors: Symbolic Action in Human Society.* Ithaca: Cornell Univ. Press, 1974.

Tyssen, Reidar, Per Maglum, Nina T. Grønvold, and Øivind Ekeberg. "Suicidal Ideation among Medical Students and Young Physicians: A Nationwide and Prospective Study of Prevalence and Predictors." *Journal of Affective Disorders* 64, no. 1 (April 2001): 69–79.

"Undergraduate Medical Education." *Journal of the American Medical Association* 234, no. 13 (29 December 1975): 1333–51.

USMLE. http://usmle.org, last accessed 1/15/08.

Van Groenou, Aneema A., and Katherine Mary Bakes. "Art, Chaos, Ethics, and Science (ACES): A Doctoring Curriculum for Emergency Medicine." *Annals of Emergency Medicine* 48, no. 5 (November 2006): 532–37.

Verghese, Abraham. *The Tennis Partner: A Doctor's Story of Friendship and Loss*. New York: HarperCollins, 1998.

———. *My Own Country: A Doctor's Story of a Town and Its People in the Age of AIDS*. New York: Simon and Schuster, 1994.

Vertosick, Frank, Jr. *When the Air Hits Your Brain*. New York: Fawcett Books, 1996.

Viscott, David S. *The Making of a Psychiatrist*. New York: Fawcett, 1972.

Waitzkin, Howard. *The Politics of Medical Encounters: How Patients and Doctors Deal with Social Problems*. New Haven: Yale Univ. Press, 1991.

Wear, Delese. "*The House of God*: Another Look." *Academic Medicine* 77, no. 6 (June 2002): 496–501.

———, Julie Aultman, Joseph D. Varley, and Joseph Zarconi. "Making Fun of Patients: Medical Students' Perceptions and Use of Derogatory and Cynical Humor in Clinical Settings." *Academic Medicine* 81, no. 5 (May 2006): 454–62.

———, Margarita Kokinova, Cynthia Keck-McNulty, and Julie Aultman. "Pimping: Perspectives of Fourth-Year Medical Students." *Teaching and Learning in Medicine* 17, no. 2 (Spring 2005): 184–91.

Whitehouse, Wayne G., David F. Dinges, Emily Carota Orne, Steven E. Keller, Brad L. Bates, Nancy K. Bauer, Page Morahan, Barbara A. Haupt, Michele M. Carlin, Peter B. Bloom, Line Zaugg, and Martin T. Orne. "Psychosocial and Immune Effects of Self-Hypnosis Training for Stress Management throughout the First Semester of Medical School." *Psychosomatic Medicine* 58, no. 3 (May–June 1996): 249–63.

Whitenton, Kristi. Kristi Whitenton's Diary. See Medschooldiary.com.

Williams, William Carlos. *The Autobiography of William Carlos Williams*. New York: New Directions, 1967.

Witte, Florence M., Terry D. Stratton, and Lois Margaret Nora. "Stories from the Field: Students' Descriptions of Gender Discrimination and Sexual Harassment during Medical School." *Academic Medicine* 81, no. 7 (July 2006): 648–54.

Wolf, T. M. "Stress, Coping, and Health: Enhancing Well-being during Medical School." *Medical Education* 28 (1994): 8–17.

X, Doctor. *Intern*. New York: Harper and Row, 1965.

Young, Audrey. *What Patients Taught Me: A Medical Student's Journey*. Seattle, WA: Sasquatch, 2004.

Index

Lewis, R. W. B., 14
Lewis, Sinclair, 14
life writing. *See* memoir
liminality, 16; in medical education, 16,
56–57, 64, 67–69, 115–16
Lovestrong. See Greenbaum, Dorothy
Ludmerer, Kenneth M., 2

MacNab, John, 59, 60, 72, 118–19, 123,
132
Maggiore, Ron, 12, 52, 59, 60, 86, 103,
128–31, 135–36, 150, 151
Making of a Psychiatrist. See Viscott,
David
Making of a Surgeon. See Nolen, William
*Making of a Surgeon in the Twenty-first
Century. See* Miller, Craig
Making of a Woman Surgeon. See Morgan,
Elizabeth
Marion, Robert, 65, 86, 88, 99–100,
113–14, 117, 119–21, 129, 142
Martin, Toni, 67–68, 88, 104, 106–07
McCarthy, Claire, 11, 64, 70, 83–84, 87,
98, 102, 116, 144
medical humanities, 4, 43, 159–66
Medical School Objectives Writing
Group (MSOP), 158–59, 166
Medschooldiary.com, 36–38
memoir, 5–9, 126–27
memoirs of medical education: in Canada,
15; narrative form and, 12–16;
representativeness of authors, 5–6; as
subgenre, 9–12
Merton, Robert K., 3
metaphor, 75–77
Miller, Craig A., 11–12, 65, 88–89, 102,
112, 136, 148–49
Miller, Jean Baker, 126
Montgomery, Kathryn, 3
Morgan, Elizabeth, 11, 49, 54, 59, 78, 89,
98, 106–09, 126, 142, 146
Morphine, Ice Cream, Tears. See Sacco,
Joseph
Mullan, Fitzhugh, 8, 53–54, 76, 81, 100

narrative competence, 165–69
Nolen, William, 11, 12, 64, 82, 88, 98–99,
121, 144–45, 146
Not Entirely Benign Procedure. See Klass,
Perri
Nuland, Sherwin B., 8
nurses: memoirs of nursing education,
82; relationship with medical students
and residents, 120–22, 148–49

Ofri, Danielle, 67, 88, 112, 116, 118, 119,
121, 128, 143
On Call. See Transue, Emily
Osborn, Claudia, 8

Parrish, John, 8
paternalism in medical education, 139
Patterson, Jane, 75, 80, 84, 101, 106, 108
physical abuse of patients, 83, 89–90,
119–22
picaresque novel, 12
Pilger, John, 9
pimping, 117
power: between patients and medical
students/residents, 115–24; theories about, 95–97. *See also* cultural
difference
practicing medical procedures on
patients, 33, 54–55
Protess, David L., 9

Rainer, J. Kenyon, 98, 100, 102, 116
reflection. *See* storytelling; writing
Reifler, Douglas R., 161–62, 164
Reilly, Philip, 12, 46, 47, 58–59, 101,
119, 128, 129–30
Reiser, Stanley Joel, 179n6
relationships in medical education, 17–
18, 125–53; with family and friends,
50, 65–66, 150–53; with patients,
25–26, 53, 54–55, 62, 70, 87–88,
129–45; with peers and colleagues, 25,
54, 60, 127–29, 145–49; with teachers,
59, 145–48